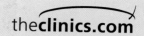

RADIOLOGIC CLINICS

OF NORTH AMERICA

Prostate Imaging

Guest Editor
PARVATI RAMCHANDANI, MD

September 2006 • Volume 44 • Number 5

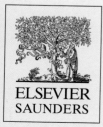

**ELSEVIER
SAUNDERS**

An imprint of Elsevier, Inc
PHILADELPHIA LONDON TORONTO MONTREAL SYDNEY TOKYO

W.B. SAUNDERS COMPANY
A Division of Elsevier Inc.

1600 John F. Kennedy Boulevard • Suite 1800 • Philadelphia, Pennsylvania 19103-2899

http://www.theclinics.com

RADIOLOGIC CLINICS OF NORTH AMERICA Volume 44, Number 5
September 2006 ISSN 0033-8389, ISBN 1-4160-3900-7

Editor: Barton Dudlick

Reprints: For copies of 100 or more, of articles in this publication, please contact the Commercial Reprints Department, Elsevier Inc., 360 Park Avenue South, New York, New York 10010-1710. Tel.: (+1) 212-633-3813; Fax: (+1) 212-462-1935; E-mail: reprints@elsevier.com.

The ideas and opinions expressed in *Radiologic Clinics of North America* do not necessarily reflect those of the Publisher does not assume any responsibility for any injury and/or damage to persons or property arising out of or related to any use of the material contained in this periodical. The reader is advised to check the appropriate medical literature and the product information currently provided by the manufacturer of each drug to be administered to verify the dosage, the method and duration of administration, or contraindications, It is the responsibility of the treating physician or other health care professional, relying on independent experience and knowledge of the patient, to determine drug dosages and the best treatment for the patient. Mention of any product in this issue should not be construed as endorsement by the contributiors, editors, or the Publisher of the productor manufacturers' claims.

Radiologic Clinics of North America (ISSN 0033-8389) is published bimonthly in January, March, May, July, September, and November by Elsevier Inc., 360 Park Avenue South, New York, NY 10010-1710. Business and editorial offices: 1600 John F. Kenedy Boulevard, Suite 1800, Philadelphia, Pennsylvania 19103-2899. Customer Service Office: 6277 Sea Harbor Drive, Orlando, FL 32887-4800. Periodicals postage paid at New York, NY, and additional mailing offices. Subscription prices are USD 259 per year for US individuals, USD 385 per year for US institutions, USD 127 per year for US students and residents, USD 303 per year for Canadian individuals, USD 473 per year of Canadian institutions, USD 352 per year for international individuals, USD 473 per year for international institutions, and USD 171 per year for Canadian and foreign students/residents. To receive student and resident rate, orders must be accompanied by name of affiliated institution, date of term, and the signature of program/residency coordinatior on institution letterhead. Orders will be billed at individual rate until proof of status is received. Foreign air speed delivery is included in all Clinics subscriptionprices. All prices are subject to change without notice. **POSTMASTER:** Send address changes to *Radiologic Clinics of North America,* Elsevier Periodicals Customer Service, 6277 Sea Harbor Drive, Orlando, FL 32887-4800. **Customer Service: 1-800-654-2452 (US). From outside of the US, call (+1) 407-345-4000.**

Radiologic Clinics of North America also published in Greek Paschalidis Medical Publications, Athens, Greece.

Radiologic Clinics of North America is covered in *Index Medicus, EMBASE/Excerpta Medica, Current Contents/Life Sciences, Current Contents/Clinical Medicine, RSNA Index to Imaging Literature, BIOSIS, Science Citation Index,* and *ISI/BIOMED.*

Printed in the United States of America.

GOAL STATEMENT

The goal of the *Radiologic Clinics of North America* is to keep practicing radiologists and radiology residents up to date with current clinical practice in radiology by providing timely articles reviewing the state of the art in patient care.

ACCREDITATION

The *Radiologic Clinics of North America* is planned and implemented in accordance with the Essential Areas and Policies of the Accreditation Council for Continuing Medical Education (ACCME) through the joint sponsorship of the University of Virginia School of Medicine and Elsevier. The University of Virginia School of Medicine is accredited by the ACCME to provide continuing medical education for physicians.

The University of Virginia School of Medicine designates this educational activity for a maximum of 15 *AMA PRA Category 1 Credits*™. Physicians should only claim credit commensurate with the extent of their participation in the activity.

The American Medical Association has determined that physicians not licensed in the US who participate in this CME activity are eligible for 15 *AMA PRA Category 1 Credits*™.

Credit can be earned by reading the text material, taking the CME examination online at http://www.theclinics.com/home/cme, and completing the evaluation. After taking the test, you will be required to review any and all incorrect answers. Following completion of the test and evaluation, your credit will be awarded and you may print your certificate.

FACULTY DISCLOSURE/CONFLICT OF INTEREST

The University of Virginia School of Medicine, as an ACCME accredited provider, endorses and strives to comply with the Accreditation Council for Continuing Medical Education (ACCME) Standards of Commercial Support, Commonwealth of Virginia statutes, University of Virginia policies and procedures, and associated federal and private regulations and guidelines on the need for disclosure and monitoring of proprietary and financial interests that may affect the scientific integrity and balance of content delivered in continuing medical education activities under our auspices.

The University of Virginia School of Medicine requires that all CME activities accredited through this institution be developed independently and be scientifically rigorous, balanced and objective in the presentation/discussion of its content, theories and practices.

All authors/editors participating in an accredited CME activity are expected to disclose to the readers relevant financial relationships with commercial entities occurring within the past 12 months (such as grants or research support, employee, consultant, stock holder, member of speakers bureau, etc.). The University of Virginia School of Medicine will employ appropriate mechanisms to resolve potential conflicts of interest to maintain the standards of fair and balanced education to the reader. Questions about specific strategies can be directed to the Office of Continuing Medical Education, University of Virginia School of Medicine, Charlottesville, Virginia.

The authors/editors listed below have identified no financial or professional relationships for themselves or their spouse/partner:
Agnieszka Szot Barnes, MD; Richard Bellah, MD; Judd Boczko, MD; Ralph Brasacchio, MD; François Cornud, MD; Vikram Dogra, MD; Barton Dudlick (Acquisitions Editor); Thomas J. Guzzo, MD; Mukesh Harisinghani, MD; Sharyn Katz, MD; Alexander Kutikov, MD; Jill E. Langer, MD; Edward Messing, MD; Andrew Mong, MD; Parvati Ramchandani, MD (Guest Editor); Mark Rosen, MD, PhD; Deborah J. Rubens, MD; John G. Strang, MD; Neil F. Wasserman, MD; and Yan Yu, PhD.

The authors/editors listed below have identified financial or professional relationships for themselves or their spouse/partner:
S. Bruce Malkowicz, MD is on the speaker's bureau for Sanofi-Aventis and Pfizer, and is an independent contractor for GTX.
Robert Ross, MD has received research grants from Astra Zeneca, Sanofi-Aventis, Genentech, and Novartis.

Disclosure of Discussion of Non-FDA Approved Uses for Pharmaceutical and/or Medical Devices.
The University of Virginia School of Medicine, as an ACCME provider, requires that all authors identify and disclose any "off label" uses for pharmaceutical and medical device products. The University of Virginia School of Medicine recommends that each physician fully review all the available data on new products or procedures prior to clinical use.

TO ENROLL

To enroll in the Radiologic Clinics of North America Continuing Medical Education program, call customer service at 1-800-654-2452 or sign up online at http://www.theclinics.com/home/cme. The CME program is available to subscribers for an additional annual fee USD 205.

FORTHCOMING ISSUE

RECENT ISSUES

PROSTATE IMAGING

GUEST EDITOR

PARVATI RAMCHANDANI, MD
Professor, Section Chief, Genitourinary Radiology,
Department of Radiology, University of
Pennsylvania Medical Center, Philadelphia,
Pennsylvania

CONTRIBUTORS

AGNIESZKA SZOT BARNES, MD
Department of Radiology, Brigham and Women's
Hospital, Boston, Massachusetts

RICHARD BELLAH, MD
Associate Professor, Department of Radiology,
The Children's Hospital of Philadelphia,
University of Pennsylvania School of Medicine,
Philadelphia, Pennsylvania

JUDD BOCZKO, MD
Department of Urology, University of Rochester
Medical Center, Rochester, New York

RALPH BRASACCHIO, MD
Department of Radiation Oncology, University
of Rochester Medical Center, Rochester, New York

FRANÇOIS CORNUD, MD
Consultant Radiologist, Hôpital Cochin,
Service de Radiologie B, Paris, France

VIKRAM DOGRA, MD
Associate Chair of Education and Research,
Professor of Radiology and Urology,
Director of Ultrasound, Director of Radiology
Residency, University of Rochester School
of Medicine, Department of Imaging Sciences,
University of Rochester Medical Center,
Rochester, New York

THOMAS J. GUZZO, MD
Clinical Instructor, Division of Urology,
Department of Surgery, University of Pennsylvania
Medical Center, Philadelphia, Pennsylvania

MUKESH HARISINGHANI, MD
Assistant Professor in Radiology, Center
for Molecular Imaging Research, Massachusetts
General Hospital, Charlestown, Massachusetts

SHARYN KATZ, MD
Instructor, Department of Radiology,
University of Pennsylvania Medical Center,
Philadelphia, Pennsylvania

ALEXANDER KUTIKOV, MD
Clinical Instructor, Division of Urology,
Department of Surgery, University
of Pennsylvania Medical Center,
Philadelphia, Pennsylvania

JILL E. LANGER, MD
Associate Professor of Radiology, Hospital
of the University of Pennsylvania, University
of Pennsylvania Medical Center, Philadelphia,
Pennsylvania

S. BRUCE MALKOWICZ, MD
Professor of Surgery, Division of Urology,
Department of Surgery, University
of Pennsylvania Medical Center,
Philadelphia, Pennsylvania

EDWARD MESSING, MD
Professor and Chairman, Department
of Urology, University of Rochester Medical
Center, Rochester, New York

ANDREW MONG, MD
Assistant Professor, Department
of Radiology, The Children's Hospital
of Philadelphia, University of Pennsylvania
School of Medicine, Philadelphia,
Pennsylvania

MARK ROSEN, MD, PhD
Assistant Professor, Department of Radiology,
University of Pennsylvania Medical Center,
Philadelphia, Pennsylvania

ROBERT ROSS, MD
Instructor in Medicine,
Dana Farber Cancer Institute, Boston;
Center for Molecular Imaging Research,
Massachusetts General Hospital, Charlestown,
Massachusetts

DEBORAH J. RUBENS, MD
Department of Imaging Sciences,
University of Rochester Medical Center,
Rochester, New York

JOHN G. STRANG, MD
Department of Imaging Sciences, University of
Rochester Medical Center, Rochester, New York

NEIL F. WASSERMAN, MD
Professor of Radiology, University of Minnesota,
Department of Veterans Affairs Medical Center,
Minneapolis, Minnesota

YAN YU, PhD
Department of Radiation Oncology, University of
Rochester Medical Center, Rochester, New York

PROSTATE IMAGING

Volume 44 · Number 5 · September 2006

Contents

Clinical Approach to the Prostate: An Update   649

Alexander Kutikov, Thomas J. Guzzo, and S. Bruce Malkowicz

> Prostatic disease continues to present clinicians with challenges. Although giant strides have been made in the medical and surgical management of benign prostatic hyperplasia, many fundamental questions about its pathogenesis, progression, and treatment efficacy remain unanswered. Prostate cancer also continues to be an area in which progress is needed despite major recent advancements. Numerous debates that include the value of prostate-specific antigen screening and the appropriate roles for each of the numerous therapeutic modalities await resolution. For millions of patients who suffer from prostatitis, a major breakthrough is yet to come. Current treatment regimens for prostatitis remain ineffective at best. Contemporary approaches to the pathogenesis, diagnosis, and treatment of benign prostatic hyperplasia, prostate cancer, and prostatitis are discussed in this review.

Inflammatory Disorders of the Prostate and the Distal Genital Tract   665

Jill E. Langer and François Cornud

> Inflammatory disease of the prostate and distal genital tract is emerging as a major health problem because it is estimated that up to 15% of adult men may be affected at some point in their lives. Clinically, the diagnosis of "prostatitis" refers to multiple disorders that cause pelvic pain and discomfort, ranging from acute bacterial infection to complex conditions that may not necessarily be caused by prostatic inflammation. Because the traditional etiology-based classification system did not always correlate with symptoms and therapeutic efficacy, a new classification of prostatitis has been suggested by the National Institutes of Health. Newer imaging techniques such as high-resolution transrectal ultrasonography (TRUS) and MR imaging provide exquisite anatomic detail and often play a crucial role in the evaluation of these patients.

postimplant assessment. Costs, availability, and ease of use often dictate the local and regional differences in imaging approach, whether ultrasound, CT, or MR. Future volumetric image developments may permit multimodality image fusion to integrate tumor-specific imaging such as MR spectrospcopy or positron emission tomography/CT into real-time ultrasound, CT, or MR.

The prostate gland is not often the target of imaging in children but may be imaged during investigation of symptoms related to the lower genitourinary tract such as hematuria, urinary retention, dysuria, and incontinence or during an evaluation for suspected congenital anomalies. Ultrasound and voiding cystourethrography are useful for initial evaluation of congenital and neoplastic disorders of the prostate. MR imaging and CT are useful in delineating more detailed anatomy before surgical planning and in determining the organ of origin in a patient who has a large pelvic mass.

RADIOLOGIC
CLINICS
OF NORTH AMERICA

Radiol Clin N Am 44 (2006) xi

Preface

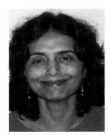

Parvati Ramchandani, MD
Guest Editor

Parvati Ramchandani, MD
Department of Radiology
University of Pennsylvania Medical Center
3400 Spruce Street
Philadelphia, PA 19104, USA

E-mail address:
ramchanp@uphs.upenn.edu

For an accessory sex gland that is normally the size of a walnut, the prostate commands much attention, both in the scientific literature and in the lay press. Anatomic parallels to the human prostate are few in mammals—dogs have a prostate that is related to the urinary bladder much as in humans, but the prostate in other mammals such as rats and nonhuman primates is very different. Both benign and malignant diseases of the prostate have few correlates in nonhuman mammals except dogs, and it remains unclear why cats, rodents, horses, and bulls, which arguably share the same environment as humans, are spared abnormal growth of the prostate. The precise function of the different accessory sex glands, such as the seminal vesicles, Cowper's gland, and the prostate—beyond contributing to the seminal ejaculate—remains unclear.

The above notwithstanding, the past decade has seen many advances in the diagnosis and treatment of prostatic diseases. Efforts remain directed at early noninvasive diagnosis and therapy that causes durable relief from the disease without a trade for unacceptable complications. I am grateful to the eminent contributors to this issue of *Radiologic Clinics of North America* who graciously expended much effort to clarify some of the most important issues relevant to the management of men with prostatic diseases. It is our hope that the readers of this issue will turn to it frequently as a valuable resource.

RADIOLOGIC
CLINICS
OF NORTH AMERICA

Radiol Clin N Am 44 (2006) 649–663

Clinical Approach to the Prostate: An Update

Alexander Kutikov, MD*, Thomas J. Guzzo, MD,
S. Bruce Malkowicz, MD

- Benign prostatic hyperplasia
  Pathophysiology
  Epidemiology
  Evaluation
  Treatment
- Adenocarcinoma of the prostate
  Epidemiology
  Risk factors
  Evaluation and screening
  Staging
  Treatment of clinically localized disease
  Therapies for advanced disease
- Prostatitis
  National Institutes of Health category I prostatitis
  National Institutes of Health category II prostatitis
  National Institutes of Health category III prostatitis
  National Institutes of Health category IV prostatitis
- Summary
- References

Embryologically, the prostate stems from the urogenital sinus. Under the influence of 5α-dihydrotestosterone (DHT), development of the gland begins at 10 weeks following fertilization. The inferior portion of the prostate (the apex) is continuous with the striated urethral sphincter. The bladder neck binds the superior portion of the gland (the base). Posteriorly and laterally, the prostate is surrounded by the capsule, a submillimeter layer of collagen, elastin, and smooth muscle. In the young adult, the prostate weighs approximately 20 g and measures $3 \times 4 \times 2$ cm [1].

The prostatic urethra, lined by transitional epithelium and enclosed in smooth muscle, hugs the anterior surface of the gland as it transverses the prostate. The urethra angulates approximately 30° anteriorly in the mid portion of the gland as it courses from the bladder to the meatus. This bend in the prostatic urethra divides it into a proximal and distal portion. The proximal portion is bound by thickened smooth muscle and is said to form the preprostatic sphincter (involuntary internal urethral sphincter). Just beyond the urethral angulation, in the early distal prostatic urethra, lies the verumontanum—a protrusion off the posterior wall of the prostatic urethra. A small aperture at the center of the verumontanum is the opening to the prostatic utricle—a vestigial Müllerian structure. Two ejaculatory ducts, a result of the union of each seminal vesicle with each vas deferens, travel approximately 2 cm from the prostatic base to the midprostatic urethra and drain to each side of the verumontanum [2].

The prostate has three distinct zones—transitional, central, and peripheral—that have different histology and distinct embryologic origins and give rise to different pathologic entities [3].

Division of Urology, Department of Surgery, University of Pennsylvania Medical Center, 9 Penn Tower, 3400 Spruce Street, Philadelphia, PA 19104, USA
* Corresponding author.
E-mail address: ak@post.harvard.edu (A. Kutikov).

doi:10.1016/j.rcl.2006.07.003

The central zone is a cone-shaped region that extends from the bladder base and encircles the ejaculatory ducts to the point of their insertion on the verumontanum. This zone is thought to be wolffian in origin and accounts for some 25% of prostatic glandular elements. The embryologic origins of this tissue may be the reason why only 1% to 5% of prostatic adenocarcinomas stem from the central zone [3].

The transitional zone surrounds the proximal (preprostatic) urethra of the prostate and, in youth, accounts for 5% to 10% of prostatic glandular tissue. This tissue is believed to be endodermal in origin and is the source of benign prostatic hypertrophy (BPH) in older men. Approximately 20% of prostate cancers arise from this zone [1,3].

The peripheral zone stems from the mesoderm and is located—as the name suggests—on the posterolateral aspect of the gland. This zone accounts for the greater part of glandular prostatic tissue and is the site of most prostatic infections. Up to 70% of prostatic adenocarcinomas arise from the peripheral zone [1,3].

The prostate contributes approximately 15% (~0.5 mL) of the ejaculatory volume. The secretions are rich in citric acid, zinc, and prostatic secretory proteins, including prostate-specific antigen (PSA). The secretion of PSA is integral in liquefaction of the semen coagulate [4].

Disorders of the prostate can be divided into three main categories: benign neoplastic, malignant neoplastic, and infectious/inflammatory pathologies. Benign neoplastic disease, known as BPH, is a widespread disorder affecting aging men, whereas adenocarcinoma of the prostate is the most common malignancy found in American men. The infectious/inflammatory diseases of the prostate are unified under the diagnosis of "prostatitis" and affect up to one third of all men at one time in their lives. Contemporary approaches to the pathogenesis, diagnosis, and treatment of these disorders are discussed in this review.

Benign prostatic hyperplasia

Benign neoplastic pathology of the prostate centers around the disease process historically referred to as prostatism, resulting in decreased force of stream, nocturia, straining, urinary frequency, and urinary urgency. Traditionally, it was believed that enlargement of the prostate (BPH) was responsible for these lower urinary tract symptoms (LUTS). It is now clear that not only glandular enlargement but also increased prostatic smooth muscle tone, decreased prostatic compliance, and altered prostatic urethral geometry can serve as culprits for LUTS. It is important to note that pathology extrinsic to the prostate, such as bladder pathology, urethral stricture disease, and bladder neck dysfunction, can also contribute to LUTS [5,6].

Pathophysiology

As a man ages, a hyperplastic process primarily of epithelial glandular tissues occurs in the transitional zone and the periurethral gland regions of the prostate. These regions enlarge by two distinct processes: an increase in the number of cells and the formation of distinct nodules [7,8]. Enlargement of the transitional zone results in hyperplasia of the "lateral lobes." This phenomenon can be clinically appreciated by observing lateral kissing tissue masses in the prostatic urethra proximal to the verumontanum on cystoscopy (albeit visual inspection by cystoscopy does not correlate well with the degree of obstruction). Obstruction of the prostatic urethra by the expanding transitional zone is believed to stem from compressive forces generated by the presence of the prostatic capsule. In canines, for instance, BPH fails to cause bladder outlet obstruction because there is no capsule combating the expansion of the transitional zone [9]. Hyperplasia of the periurethral glands at the bladder neck in some individuals gives rise to the "median lobe," a tissue mass that can ball-valve into the bladder neck and cause significant obstructing symptoms. Moreover, a noteworthy share of outlet obstruction generated by the prostate on the bladder outlet is thought to be due to the intrinsic prostatic urethral resistance, mediated by the α_{1a} receptors [10–13]. This latter observation has paved the way for one of the primary medical treatment options of BPH. Specific changes in gene expression, cellular morphology, and molecular signaling have been examined and implicated in the pathogenesis of BPH [14]. The multifaceted interaction between anatomic and physiologic factors makes BPH pathophysiology a complex and still poorly understood process that transcends the simplistic notion of bulky prostate size causing obstruction.

Epidemiology

Assessment of the prevalence and incidence of BPH pivots on how the disease is defined. When a histologic definition is applied and autopsy series are examined, 50% of men in the fifth decade of life demonstrate evidence of BPH [15]. Histologic prevalence of BPH, however, is less clinically relevant than the prevalence of symptomatic disease. One of the largest studies conducted to date assessed the LUTS severity in 7588 men from nine Asian countries. Investigators demonstrated that 18% of men in their 40s, 29% of men in their 50s, 40% of men in their 60s, and 56% of men in their 70s had LUTS. These rates are similar to the prevalence of LUTS in Australia, America, and Europe [16].

Evaluation

Evaluation of a patient who has LUTS indicative of BPH begins with obtaining a medical history. History of conditions contributing to bladder dysfunction and polyuria must be elicited. Past medical history and family history of BPH and prostate cancer should also be obtained. To best assess patient symptomatology at presentation and to appropriately follow response to treatment, LUTS should be quantified using the American Urologic Association (AUA) Symptom Index (AUA-SI; an identical questionnaire to the International Prostate Symptom Score). The seven questions of the AUA-SI assess frequency, nocturia, weak urinary stream, hesitancy, intermittence, incomplete emptying, and urgency [17].

A physical examination should be preformed and must include a digital rectal examination (DRE) [5]. DRE has been shown to underestimate prostate size; however, it is useful in identifying very large prostates because the glands that feel oversized on DRE usually prove to be hyperplastic on transrectal ultrasound [18]. DRE is also useful to assess for presence of locally invasive prostate cancer because this may be the etiology of LUTS in an elderly man [19]. A focused neurologic examination to evaluate mental status, lower extremity neuromuscular function, and sphincter tone is also often performed [5].

Bladder cancer, bladder calculi, and urinary tract infections can all cause LUTS. Urinalysis (a screen for hematuria and urinary tract infections) is therefore recommended in men who present with LUTS. For those men who have principally irritative voiding symptoms or a strong history of smoking or industrial exposures, a voided urine cytology specimen may be considered to evaluate for presence of bladder cancer [5].

A discussion about PSA screening should take place with patients undergoing evaluation for LUTS suggestive of BPH. PSA levels in patients who have BPH have been shown to be a predictor of symptom progression, spontaneous acute urinary retention, and future prostate growth [5,20–23]. In combination with DRE, PSA can serve as a useful tool to exclude locally invasive prostate cancer as the source of the LUTS [5]. Nevertheless, some 25% of BPH patients will have a PSA level greater than 4 ng/mL, necessitating a prostate needle biopsy. Patients must be made aware of this nonspecific nature of PSA testing.

Uroflowmetry and postvoid residual determination are often performed at the initial evaluation of patients who have LUTS; however, these evaluations are not mandatory because guideline values of maximum flow rate and postvoid residual volumes for management decision making have not been established [5].

Historically, serum creatinine values were routinely obtained for patients who had LUTS. This practice is now considered unnecessary because patients who have BPH have been shown to have the same rates of renal insufficiency as the general population (under 1%) [5].

Treatment

After patients who have LUTS have undergone the necessary workup, a discussion must take place regarding the risks and benefits of watchful waiting, medical management, or surgical intervention.

Watchful waiting

Patients who have an AUA-SI score of 7 or less are said to have mild symptoms and are primary candidates for watchful waiting. Watchful waiting is also appropriate for men who have more severe LUTS, are reluctant to initiate life-long medical or invasive surgical therapies, and do not exhibit signs of BPH complications such as urinary tract infections, renal insufficiency, bladder stones, or urinary retention. Reassurance and simple intervention such as reduced fluid ingestion before going to sleep and limited alcohol and caffeine intake can successfully manage these patients [24]. The principal question that arises when patients are placed on watchful waiting is whether a delay in intervention poses risks to the patient. To date, this question remains largely unanswered. Concerns about bladder decompensation are worrisome but remain theoretic; however, limited data exist that show that patients who are initially treated with watchful waiting may do less well than those in whom intervention is undertaken. One prospective study randomized men who had moderate LUTS to watchful waiting or to transurethral resection of the prostate (TURP). After 5 years of follow-up, men who crossed over into the TURP treatment arm after a trial of watchful waiting had the same rate of serious adverse outcomes and general degree of bother from LUTS as men who were resected immediately, but the former group failed to show the same level of improvement in symptom score and flow rate [25]. Nevertheless, experts agree that watchful waiting is generally a safe approach [5,24,26,27]. Reevaluation of patients placed on watchful waiting should take place at least annually [5].

Medical therapy

In the last 20 years, there has been a paradigm shift in BPH treatment. Immediate treatment with surgical intervention has given way to medical therapy. Two major drug classes are employed in management of LUTS secondary to BPH: α-adrenergic blockers and 5α-reductase inhibitors.

α-Adrenergic blockers As discussed previously, intrinsic prostatic urethral resistance, mediated by the α_{1a} receptors, contributes significantly to bladder outlet obstruction resulting from BPH [10]. Inhibition of the α_{1a} receptors by oral agents such as alfuzosin, doxazosin, tamsulosin, and terazosin has been shown to reduce the AUA-SI by an average of 4 to 6 points within weeks of initiation of therapy [5,24,28]. A meta-analysis by the AUA guideline panel of these four agents established them as therapeutically equivalent [5]. Because of this similarity in therapeutic efficacy, in the current era, the choice between the available agents is based on ease of administration, the relevance of the agent's side-effect profile to a given patient, and cost. For instance, treatment with tamsulosin—a highly selective α_{1a} receptor antagonist—is associated with ease of administration and a low incidence of orthostatic hypotension but a high incidence of retrograde ejaculation and higher costs [5]. Overall, the α-adrenergic blockers are associated with relatively mild side effects that include dizziness, headache, fatigue, postural hypotension, nasal congestion, edema, and retrograde ejaculation [6,29]. The first-line use of α-adrenergic blockers in the treatment of BPH has become common for the primary care physician and the urologist.

5α-Reductase inhibitors A second major class of drugs employed in the management of BPH is the 5α-reductase isoenzyme inhibitors. As discussed earlier, the embryologic development of the prostate is androgen dependent and driven by DHT. Androgens continue to play a role in prostatic volume maintenance in adult life. This was well documented at the end of the nineteenth century when surgical castration was noted to reduce prostate size [30]. Because 90% of testosterone is converted to DHT within the prostate, selective inhibition of this conversion of testosterone to its more potent counterpart reduces prostate size and affects LUTS in men who have BPH while maintaining serum testosterone levels within the normal range [31]. The 5α-reductase enzymes catalyze the reduction of testosterone to DHT. Two isoenzymes exist. The liver, sebaceous glands, skin, and most hair follicles express the Type 1 isoenzyme, whereas the Type 2 isoform is present in the skin of the genitalia, facial/scalp hair follicles, and the prostate (some Type 1 isoenzyme may also be present) [31,32]. Finasteride is a competitive inhibitor of the Type 2 isoenzyme. It is estimated that the agent causes a 65% to 70% reduction in serum and an 85% to 90% reduction in the prostatic DHT levels [31,33]. With finasteride therapy, prostatic glandular epithelium atrophies and prostate size decreases by 15% to 30% within several months [6,34]. Dutasteride, a newcomer to the BPH scene, inhibits Type 1 and Type 2 enzymes, resulting in a more global suppression of DHT than finasteride [35]. Randomized head-to-head studies of dutasteride and finasteride have not yet been performed, but the agents appear to be clinically identical [5,31]. An average reduction of 3 points on the AUA-SI occurs with 5α-reductase treatment—less than for α-adrenergic blockade. Finasteride has been found ineffective in men who have normal-sized prostates, and the AUA guidelines for the management of BPH do not recommend 5α-reductase treatment in these patients [5,36]. The onset of action is generally unhurried, taking up to 6 months, but appears to be consequential, blocking prostatic growth and resulting in some 50% reduction in the rate of urinary retention and the need for surgical intervention [22,34,35,37–39]. 5α-Reductase treatment is well tolerated but carries a small risk of libido reduction and erectile dysfunction [31,34].

Combination therapy Given the very distinct mechanisms of action of 5α-reductase inhibitors and α-adrenergic blockers, synergistic or at least additive action is expected. Initial clinical trials, 1 year or less in duration, combined the two agents and enrolled men who had relatively small glands. No benefit of adding a 5α-reductase inhibitor to an α-adrenergic blocker could be shown in these studies [40,41]. A more recent large, randomized, placebo-controlled, double-blind trial was reported [42]. This trial enrolled 3047 men at least 50 years old with a mean prostate volume of 36.3 cm^3 (SD, 20.1 cm^3) and an AUA-SI of 8 to 30 (mean, 16.9). These patients were randomized to placebo, doxazosin, finasteride, or combination therapy. The mean length of follow-up was 4.5 years, and the patients were monitored for clinical BPH progression. Disease progression was defined as at least a 4-point rise in the AUA-SI, acute urinary retention, urinary incontinence, renal insufficiency, or recurrent urinary tract infections. In the placebo arm, 17% of men were noted to have progression of BPH, with most (80%) demonstrating a 4-point or greater increase in the AUA-SI score. Only 10% of patients showed disease progression in the doxazosin-treated arm (39% risk reduction). Similar results were seen in the finasteride-treated patients (34% reduction). The combination therapy group demonstrated a cumulative incidence of progression of only 5% (a reduction of 66%). This reduction with combination therapy was significantly greater ($P < .001$) than with finasteride or doxazosin alone [42]. Based on these data, most urologists currently choose combination therapy for patients who have significant LUTS and documented prostatic enlargement. Patients who have relatively small prostates, on the other hand, are treated with α-adrenergic blockade monotherapy [39].

Surgical therapy

Indications for surgical therapy for BPH include urinary retention, intractable LUTS, recurrent urinary tract infections, azotemia, or recurrent hematuria. In today's practice, many procedures are performed for patients who have been placed on medical management but continue to suffer moderate to severe LUTS.

Open prostatectomy   Surgical treatment of BPH was born in the late nineteenth century when open prostatectomy was pioneered [6]. Open prostatectomy for BPH involves enucleation of the periurethral prostatic tissues, leaving the prostatic capsule intact. A retropubic or a suprapubic approach can be employed. Retropubic prostatectomy (RP) involves making a lower abdominal incision and gaining access to the adenoma through an incision in the anterior prostatic capsule. Suprapubic (also known as transvesical) prostatectomy achieves the same result through an extraperitoneal incision in the anterior bladder wall. The latter approach is reserved for patients who have large median lobes or concurrent bladder calculi. In the current era, open benign prostatectomy is limited to glands greater than 100 cm^3 and, therefore, performed in less than 1% of patients who have BPH [5,6,43]. New evidence, however, suggests that open prostatectomy should continue to be a viable option for patients who have BPH because the reoperation rate is low and the morbidity is comparable to TURP [44].

Transurethral resection of the prostate   TURP is said to be the hallmark of the urologist and is the "gold standard" for BPH treatment [6,45]. Prostatic adenoma is resected transurethrally using an electrocautery loop. Hemostasis is achieved with the same instrument, and no abdominal incisions are necessary. The procedure is performed under general or spinal anesthesia. Because absorptive hyponatremia (TURP syndrome) occurs in some 2% of patients undergoing TURP, spinal anesthesia is preferred. Hyponatremia results in vision disturbances along with changes in mental status, and this can be easily monitored under spinal anesthesia during the resection [46]. As stated previously, TURP remains the benchmark by which all other treatments are compared. Nearly 90% of patients undergoing TURP see an improvement in their symptom score. The reduction in the symptom score is profound. When expressed as the percentage improvement with respect to the pretreatment AUA-SI score

([AUA-SI score before TURP − AUA-SI score after TURP] × 100/AUA-SI score before TURP), a reduction that exceeds 80% is observed [47]. The Veterans Affairs Cooperative Study is the most authoritative clinical investigation evaluating TURP. Wasson and colleagues [26] conducted a multicenter, prospective, randomized trial of TURP versus watchful waiting. Patients who had a mean AUA-SI score of 14.6 were randomized to TURP or watchful waiting. During the follow-up of 3 years, these men were monitored for treatment failure. Treatment failure was defined as death, repeated or persistent urinary retention, postvoid residual of 350 mL or greater, development of bladder stones, incontinence, a high AUA-SI score (≥21 twice or ≥24 once), or doubling of the serum creatinine concentration. Treatment failure was found to be twice as likely in the watchful-waiting group (3.0 per 100 person years) than in the TURP group (6.1 per 100 person years). This difference was highly statistically significant (P = .002). An average reduction of 9.6 AUA-SI points was noted in the TURP group (compared with −5.5 in the watchful waiting group, $P < .001$). Men also reported a significant improvement in bother from urinary difficulties and in activities of daily living. Best outcomes from TURP were seen in those patients who were highly bothered by urinary symptoms at baseline. This study put into question the urologic dogma, derived from retrospective observations, that men undergoing TURP are at a risk for incontinence and erectile dysfunction—no difference was seen between the surgery and the watchful-waiting arms.

Laser therapy   Ablation of prostatic tissue with laser energy has gained momentum during the last decade. After initial disappointment with Nd:YAG visual laser ablation of the prostate in the early 1990s, technologic advances have thrust laser treatments to the frontlines of surgical interventions for BPH. One of the best studied laser modalities is the holmium:YAG laser enucleation of the prostate (HoLEP). Employing the retrograde urethral approach, the median and lateral lobes of the prostate are enucleated from the prostatic capsule using a front-firing laser-emitting fiber. The prostatic tissue is pushed into the bladder and then extracted with specially designed evacuators/morcillators. In several comparative studies, symptom relief was identical in patients who underwent HoLEP and TURP at 6 and 12 months postoperatively [48]. HoLEP's superb success against urinary retention was also recently demonstrated [49]. The technique is generally more time consuming than a standard TURP, but shorter catheterization time and hospital stays have been consistently documented [48,50].

The procedure is technically demanding, and it is estimated that performing up to 25 cases is required to acquire competence [51]. This main disadvantage of HoLEP has limited its popularity.

The laser prostatectomy technique that has gained widespread appeal among urologists and patients in the recent years is the potassium titanyl phosphate (KTP) laser prostatectomy. Also known as the photoselective vaporization of the prostate (PVP) or the GreenLight prostatectomy, this surgical approach removes prostatic tissue employing a side-firing KTP laser-emitting fiber. The procedure is easy to learn and produces a TURP-like defect in the prostatic tissues [50–52]. The coagulating properties of the KTP laser stem from the strong absorption of this wavelength (532 nm) by hemoglobin, and make the technique an attractive option for patients who cannot tolerate blood loss or stop anticoagulation therapy [52,53]. More data are needed to define the technique's long-term efficacy, but its safety and ease of use has firmly established PVP's foothold in the urologist's armamentarium [54].

A competing technique, holmium laser ablation of the prostate, is a method similar to PVP that harnesses the vaporizing properties of the holmium: YAG laser [55]. Long-term data now exist for this approach when a maximum average power of 60 W is employed. At this energy, the technique is safe but time-consuming and tedious because the holmium:YAG laser does not penetrate tissue as deeply as the KTP wavelength. The new 100-W power holmium:YAG laser has been introduced to the market and holds more promise, increasing the technique's vaporization efficiency [55].

The urologic community still awaits prospective randomized trials comparing the various techniques for the laser ablation of the prostate.

Thermal therapy Transurethral microwave thermotherapy (TUMT) for BPH produces coagulation necrosis of prostatic tissues through heat produced by a microwave-emitting coil. Several companies produce devices that work in a similar manner. Most employ a high-energy source coupled with a water-cooling balloon that assures safe temperatures in the prostatic urethra [56]. TUMT therapy is safe and effective in the short-term but is plagued by prolonged irritative voiding symptoms and post-treatment urinary retention. Effectiveness of TUMT is consistently inferior to TURP in randomized trials. Based on available evidence, the AUA guidelines on management of BPH view TUMT as superior to medical therapy but inferior to surgical options [5,56].

Transurethral needle ablation of the prostate (TUNA) is a therapy that, like TUMP, employs heat to produce coagulation necrosis in the lateral lobes of the prostate. Heating of prostate tissue is achieved with two radiofrequency energy–emitting 18-guage needles that protrude from the tip of the TUNA catheter [57]. Clinically, TUNA is very similar to TUMT, resulting in symptom relief that appears to surpass medical therapy but falls short of TURP. Irritative voiding symptoms and transient urinary retention are also common following TUNA treatment. TUNA and TUMP are outpatient office procedures, but TUNA seems to require more analgesia [5].

Adenocarcinoma of the prostate

Epidemiology

Adenocarcinoma of the prostate is the most common noncutaneous malignancy in the Western world [58,59]. Prostate cancer accounts for 12% of the total cancer prevalence [60]. There will be a projected 234,460 new cases of prostate cancer diagnosed in the United States in 2006, with an estimated 27,350 deaths [58,61]. The incidence of prostate cancer has dramatically risen over the past 2 decades largely due to the implementation of widespread PSA screening [58,62]. The impact of PSA screening on prostate cancer–specific mortality is less clear. Although prostate cancer mortality rates have declined over the last decade, there is not yet definitive evidence to link PSA screening to this decrease in mortality. Two large randomized clinical trials (the European Randomized Study of Screening for Prostate Cancer Trial and the Prostate, Lung, Colorectal, and Ovary Cancer Trial) are presently ongoing in an attempt to answer this question.

Risk factors

There are several well-defined risk factors for the development of prostate cancer. Prostate cancer rates vary widely among ethnic groups, with African American men having the highest incidence of prostate cancer in the United States (170 cases per 100,000 men in 1995) compared with Asian American men who have the low incidence of prostate cancer (82 cases per 100,000 men in 1995) [58,63]. Endogenous androgen levels are generally higher in African Americans than in Caucasians, and these higher levels have been postulated to play a role in the development of prostate cancer [64]. The incidence of prostate cancer in Caucasian and Hispanic American men is 104 and 82 per 100,000 men, respectively [63].

Prostate cancer rates are also quite variable geographically throughout the world. The United States, Canada, and Scandinavia have a relatively high incidence of prostate cancer compared with countries such as Japan and China [58,63].

As men age, the risk of developing prostate cancer increases. Prostate cancer has been found incidentally in approximately 30% of autopsy specimens of men in their sixth decade [58,61]. Seventy percent to 80% of patients who have prostate cancer are older than 65 years [58,64]. Prostate cancer is a rare finding in men under age 45 years, with an incidence of 0.4 in 100,000 per year [65].

A family history of prostate cancer is a significant risk for the development of prostate cancer. Men who have one first-degree relative who has prostate cancer have a twofold risk of developing prostate cancer. This risk increases with more affected first-degree relatives such that men who have two or three first-degree relatives with prostate cancer have a fivefold or an 11-fold risk of developing prostate cancer, respectively [66]. True hereditary prostate cancer accounts for a small number of prostate cancer cases. As described by Carter and colleagues [67], hereditary prostate cancer is defined as cancer in three consecutive generations, a cluster of three first-degree relatives, or two relatives affected before age 55 years. Several genes are currently being investigated for their role in the genetic inheritance of prostate cancer [58,68].

Diets high in animal fat have also been associated with a risk of prostate cancer [69,70]. It has also been shown that immigrants to Western cultures from Japan and China develop prostate cancer at an incidence equaling their new culture [70,71]. Although there is contradictory evidence it the literature, an association between diet and prostate cancer appears to be real. Conversely, several dietary agents have been postulated to have a protective effect on the development of prostate cancer, including lycopene, soy products, zinc, selenium, and vitamin E [70].

Evaluation and screening

Early prostate cancers demonstrate few signs and symptoms given that most of these cancers develop in the peripheral portion of the prostate. The presence of symptoms such as hematuria, obstructive voiding symptoms, and bone pain generally indicate the presence of advanced disease. Clinically localized disease is usually suspected based on an elevated PSA or abnormal DRE, prompting transrectal ultrasound–guided biopsy of the prostate for definitive diagnosis.

The widespread use of PSA testing has led to a dramatic increase in the number of cases of clinically localized prostate cancer over the last 2 decades [62]. PSA is a 240–amino acid serine protease coded for on chromosome 19 and is a member of the human kallikrein gene family [72]. The functional role of PSA is not entirely understood, but PSA is secreted in high concentrations in the seminal fluid whereby it acts to liquefy the seminal coagulum. PSA is found in much lower concentrations in the serum where it exists in bound and unbound forms [73]. The bound form is more common, and PSA is generally found complexed to the antiproteases alpha$_1$-antichymotrypsin or alpha$_2$-macroglobulin [74]. The generally excepted normal serum value for PSA is 4.0 ng/mL or less. Elevated serum PSA levels can be due to a variety of factors including prostate cancer, ejaculation, prostatic inflammation and infection, BPH, and recent urologic instrumentation [75].

The impact of PSA screening on prostate cancer survival remains controversial. There are several prospective, randomized, controlled trials currently underway to answer this question. The American Cancer Society and the AUA recommend prostate cancer screening consisting of annual DRE and serum PSA starting at age 50 years for all men who have a life expectancy of greater than 10 years and at age 40 years for African American men or men who have a family history of prostate cancer. The most effective form of prostate cancer screening is the use of PSA and DRE together [76]. The exact "cutoff" value for an abnormal PSA value remains controversial. Generally, a serum value of less than 4.0 ng/mL is accepted as normal, but more recently, a PSA cutoff of 2.5 ng/mL in men younger than 60 years has been suggested [77]. It has also been noted that an absolute PSA value may not be as important as PSA velocity. Multiple studies suggest that if the serum PSA increases greater than 0.75 ng/mL per year, there is a significant risk for prostate cancer regardless of the absolute serum PSA value [78].

When a patient has been identified on screening with an abnormal DRE or PSA, generally the next step is transrectal ultrasound–guided prostate needle biopsy. The use of transrectal ultrasound alone has proved to be unreliable in detecting prostate cancer; thus, all patients should undergo biopsy regardless of the ultrasound findings [79]. Over the years, the number of biopsy samples and their location have undergone numerous revisions, but studies have shown that an increased number of biopsy samples from the traditional sextant biopsy scheme has improved cancer detection and decreased the number of false-negative results [80]. Transrectal ultrasound–guided prostate biopsy is generally well tolerated by patients in the office setting. The most common complications cited are hematuria, hematospermia, and hematochezia. These findings are generally self-limiting and resolve in days to weeks. Severe complications including severe bleeding, sepsis, and urinary retention occur in less than 5% of cases [81].

Staging

It is well documented that the pathologic stage of prostate cancer directly affects prognostic outcome [82]. Clinical staging is used as a systematic and clinically proven way to predict prognosis and direct treatment. The primary resources used to clinically stage patients who have prostate cancer are DRE, serum PSA, histologic tumor grading, and radiographic studies.

DRE is used to estimate local tumor extent. The sensitivity and specificity of DRE to predict organ-confined disease is low [83]. Studies have demonstrated significant understaging of prostate cancer by DRE [84]. PSA is a useful tumor marker to aid the clinician in predicting clinical stage in patients who have prostate cancer. Serum PSA levels have been shown to positively correlate with pathologic stage and tumor volumes [85]. Eighty percent of men who have serum PSA values less than 4.0 ng/mL will have organ-confined disease [86]. It has also been demonstrated that two thirds of men who have prostate cancer whose serum PSA is between 4 and 10 ng/mL have organ-confined disease and that greater than 50% of men who have serum PSA levels greater than 10 ng/mL have disease not confined to the prostate [86].

The Gleason grading system is the most widely excepted histologic grading system for prostate cancer [87]. This system is based on the microscopic description of the prostatic adenocarcinoma. A Gleason pattern of 1 to 5 (1 being the lowest grade and 5 being the highest grade) is assigned to primary and secondary areas of prostate cancer in a biopsy specimen. These two grades, added together, determine the Gleason score. Multiple well-designed studies have demonstrated the usefulness of Gleason scoring to predict prognosis of patients who have prostate cancer. The presence of Gleason grade 7 disease or greater is predictive of a poor prognosis and a higher likelihood of biochemical failure after definitive treatment for prostate cancer [88]. Partin and colleagues [89] constructed probability tables using preoperative serum PSA, clinical stage, and Gleason score to predict the pathologic stage of prostate cancer. These tables have proved to be invaluable in counseling patients about treatment options and prognosis.

Imaging modalities such as bone scanning, abdominal and pelvic CT scanning, and endorectal MR imaging have also been employed in an attempt to further stratify patients before definitive therapy. Bone scanning is the most sensitive radiographic test to diagnose bony metastases [90]. In patients who have a PSA of less than 10 ng/mL, the chance of finding metastatic prostate cancer on a bone scan is approximately 0.1%. Cross-sectional imaging to evaluate for the presence of local extension and lymphadenopathy has a low sensitivity and is not recommended [91]. More recently, MR imaging with an endorectal coil has been used in an attempt to provide additional staging information, but most studies to date have not demonstrated a beneficial affect [92].

The most commonly used pathologic staging system for prostate cancer is the TNM staging system. Table 1 outlines the most recent American Joint Committee on Cancer TNM staging system [93].

Treatment of clinically localized disease

Multiple therapeutic strategies are available to men who have clinically localized prostate cancer, including radical surgery, external beam radiation, prostate brachytherapy, cryosurgery, and watchful waiting with or without hormonal ablative therapy. The type of therapy employed depends on multiple factors including patient age and life expectancy, comorbid conditions, willingness to accept the potential complications of treatment, and patient preference.

Watchful waiting

Watchful waiting for patients who have prostate cancer is generally used as an alternative to definitive treatment in patients who have a life expectancy of less than 10 years. The goal of this approach is to manage the disease expectantly, with the initiation of palliative therapies as progression occurs. More recently, the concept of expectant management with curative intent has been employed by some centers [94]. The rational for this approach stems from the fact that increasing numbers of older men are being diagnosed with prostate cancer as the result of PSA screening. Given the fact the treatment of older men who have low-grade disease is unlikely to affect their life span, these patients are managed expectantly until the first sign of disease progression, at which point active therapy is instituted [95]. Early data have shown that this approach may be a reasonable alternative to definitive treatment in older men who have prostate cancer [94].

Radical surgery

The "gold standard" for treatment of men who have clinically localized prostate cancer with a life expectancy of 10 years or greater remains radical RP. Although radical RP is performed in most open surgeries for prostate cancer, the perineal approach is still used in a small subset of patients. RP is generally reserved for patients who have clinically localized disease (stage T1–T2). RP involves removal of the prostate with reanstamosis of the bladder

Table 1: **Prostate Cancer TNM American Joint Committee on Cancer staging system, 2002**

Stage	Description
TX	Primary tumor cannot be assessed
T1	Clinically inapparent tumor not palpable or visible by imaging
T1a	Normal DRE; incidental tumor < 5% of TURP specimen, Gleason score < 7
T1b	Normal DRE; incidental tumor > 5% of TURP specimen, Gleason score $\geq$ 7
T1c	Normal DRE; tumor diagnosed on prostate needle biopsy for elevated PSA
T2	Tumor confined to prostate
T2a	Organ confined, tumor limited to half of one lobe of prostate
T2b	Organ confined, tumor confined to more than half of one lobe but not both lobes
T2c	Organ confined, tumor involving both lobes of prostate
T3	Tumor extending through prostate capsule
T3a	Extracapsular extension (unilateral or bilateral)
T3b	Tumor invading seminal vesicle (unilateral or bilateral)
T4	Tumor fixed or invades adjacent structures other than seminal vesicles
NX	Regional lymph nodes cannot be assessed
N0	No regional lymph node metastasis
N1	Metastasis in regional lymph node or nodes
MX	Distant metastasis cannot be assessed
M0	No distant metastasis
M1a	Nonregional lymph node metastasis
M1b	Bone metastasis
M1c	Other metastatic sites with or without bone disease

to the proximal urethra, with or without a pelvic lymph node dissection. As more and more men are undergoing RP secondary to PSA screening, a greater emphasis has been placed on surgical morbidity and postsurgical quality of life. The most common complications after radical prostatectomy include impotence, incontinence, and bladder neck contracture [96]. Identification of the nerves to the penile corpora and description of the anatomic radical prostatectomy by Walsh and Donker [97] has dramatically decreased the morbidity associated with this operation. Now with "nerve-sparing procedures," the incidence of impotence after radical prostatectomy is far less than in older series. Generally with a nerve-sparing procedure, younger men and men who had good-quality erections before surgery have the greatest chance of maintaining function after surgery [98]. The 5-year progression-free survival rate after radical prostatectomy approaches 80% regardless of tumor stage or Gleason score. In patients who have Gleason grade 6 organ-confined disease, the 10-year biochemical progression-free survival rate is between 91% and 97% [82,98].

Over the last several years, minimally invasive approaches to radical prostatectomy have gained popularity. Laparoscopic radical prostatectomy from a transperitoneal and an extraperitoneal approach has been described. Robotic prostatectomy is also gaining popularity at several specialized centers across the country. The benefits of these "minimally invasive" approaches are a quicker recovery time, a smaller incision, less intraoperative blood loss, and potentially less incidence of postsurgical impotence and incontinence. Although preliminary data appear promising, long-term data are lacking [99–101].

Brachytherapy

Brachytherapy for prostate cancer involves the placement of radioactive seeds by way of a transperineal approach directly into the prostate. The two isotopes most commonly used for implantation are iodine 125 and palladium 103. Generally, brachytherapy is most effective in patients who have lower-grade cancers (Gleason biopsy score <7, PSA <10 ng/mL, and stage T1–T2) [102]. In low-risk patients, brachytherapy has been shown to have outcomes similar to radical prostatectomy and external beam radiation [102]. Side effects of brachytherapy include urinary retention, worsening or new onset of LUTS, urethral stricture, impotence, diarrhea, rectal mucosal ulceration, and rectal bleeding [103].

External beam radiation

External beam radiation can be used as a definitive treatment for clinically localized prostate cancer and is widely accepted as the treatment of choice in men who have clinically advanced disease [104,105]. External beam radiation is traditionally administered in divided doses of 70 to 80 Gy.

Newer methods of delivering radiation to the prostate, including CT-based treatment planning and three-dimensional conformational radiation therapy, have improved the accuracy of delivering radiation to the prostate while limiting unwarranted radiation to surrounding tissues. Side effects related to external beam radiation include diarrhea, radiation proctitis, impotence, skin reactions, hematuria, and hemorrhagic cystitis [106].

Cryotherapy

Cryotherapy for prostate cancer is performed by using cryoprobes that are inserted directly into the prostate by way of the transperineal approach. Cellular injury occurs due to freezing and thawing, which directly kills cells. Cryotherapy, like brachytherapy, is more suitable for patients who have low-risk prostate cancer [107].

Therapies for advanced disease

Hormonal therapy

Hormonal ablation has been used in men who have advanced prostate cancer. The exact timing of when to institute therapy remains controversial. In general, hormonal ablation can limit or relieve symptoms secondary to prostate cancer and can prolong time to clinical progression, but it is debatable weather hormonal therapy prolongs survival [108]. Hormonal ablation can be achieved in several ways including surgical castration or medical castration. Advantages of bilateral orchiectomy include immediate onset of action, "one time" cost, and lack of compliance issues. A number of medications are available to suppress circulating androgens to castration levels. Estrogens, leutenizing hormone–releasing hormone agonists, and direct antiandrogen blocking medications have been used. The benefits from the institution of androgen blockade, whether medical or surgical, must be weighed against the potential side effects including loss of libido, erectile dysfunction, anemia, hot flashes, loss of muscle mass, and loss of bone density [109].

Chemotherapy

Historically, chemotherapy for the treatment of hormone refractory prostate cancer has been reserved for the treatment of severe bone pain. Recently, docetaxel-based therapy has demonstrated an extension in survival for men who have hormone refractory metastatic prostate cancer [110]. The promising results from the docetaxel trials have provided renewed interest for the potential treatment of advanced prostate cancer with chemotherapeutic agents.

Prostatitis

The infectious and inflammatory pathology of the prostate is encompassed by the clinical entity known as prostatitis. It is estimated that some 30% men will suffer from prostatitis-like symptoms at some point in life. Less than 10% of patients, however, will ever have any documented evidence of infection [111]. Four subtypes of prostatitis are described by the National Institutes of Health (NIH) classification [112]:

NIH category I—acute bacterial prostatitis
NIH category II—chronic bacterial prostatitis
NIH category III—chronic prostatitis/chronic pelvic pain syndrome (CP/CPPS)
IIIA—inflammatory
IIIB—noninflammatory
NIH category IV—asymptomatic inflammatory (incidentally found on biopsy)

Acute and chronic bacterial prostatitis are the most infrequent but the best characterized prostatitis subtypes, whereas category III prostatitis is the most widespread entity but still poorly understood [112]. Category IV disease is by definition asymptomatic and appears to be an extraneous clinical entity.

National Institutes of Health category I prostatitis

Acute bacterial prostatitis is an uncommon infectious process of the male urinary tract. Infectious culprits are most often gram-negative uropathogens that are believed to seed the prostate through the prostatic ducts by way of reflux [113]. Patients who have NIH category I prostatitis are acutely ill and can present with fevers, elevated leukocyte counts, complaints of suprapubic, perineal or genital pain, urinary retention, and even septic shock. Physical examination reveals an exquisitely tender prostate. The possibility of a prostatic abscess should always be considered and evaluated with CT scan or a transrectal ultrasound. Treatment involves antibiotic therapy and drainage of an abscess if present.

National Institutes of Health category II prostatitis

Chronic bacterial prostatitis is a very rare clinical entity that is found in men who have recurrent cystitis. Between the episodes of cystitis, bacteria can be cultured from prostatic secretions following prostatic massage. A prolonged course of lipophilic antibiotics such as trimethoprim-sulfamethoxazole or fluoroquinolones is indicated because these antimicrobial agents achieve high concentrations in prostatic tissues. Chronic suppressive antibiotic therapy can be used for patients who continue to have documented episodes of prostatitis despite initial treatment [114].

National Institutes of Health category III prostatitis

Chronic prostatitis/chronic pelvic pain syndrome (CP/CPPS) accounts for greater than 90% of clinically encountered prostatitis. Patients in the IIIA subtype exhibit leukocytes in their prostatic secretions (but no infection), whereas NIH category IIIB patients reveal no evidence of inflammation [112]. CP/CPPS is a symptoms complex that is poorly understood and may stem from nonprostatic pathology in some patients [115]. CP/CPPS patients suffer from a compilation of nonspecific complaints that can be divided into four categories: (1) pain symptoms—perineal, penile, suprapubic, anal, and pelvic pain, and testicular discomfort; (2) voiding symptoms—dysuria, urinary frequency, urgency, and poor stream; (3) sexual dysfunction—pain on ejaculation and erectile difficulties; and (4) generic symptoms—backache, fatigue, and malaise [113]. Treatment of CP/CPPS continues to be a frustrating exercise for the patient and the physician. Antibiotic therapy, α-adrenergic blockers, anti-inflammatory agents, muscle relaxants, and minimally invasive surgical techniques are often used to treat the condition but result in modest to no benefit [116,117]. It is unfortunate that few improved treatment options are on the horizon [118].

National Institutes of Health category IV prostatitis

NIH category IV inflammatory prostatitis is by definition found in asymptomatic men and is a histologic diagnosis made on prostate biopsy. The diagnosis can also be made from (1) prostate chips from TURP or (2) prostatic secretions of asymptomatic men. No treatment is indicated for this clinically insignificant entity. Some clinicians advise a course of fluoroquinolones in men who have NIH category IV prostatitis and an elevated PSA.

Summary

Prostatic disease continues to present clinicians with challenges. Giant strides have been made in the medical and surgical management of BPH; however, many fundamental questions about pathogenesis, progression, and treatment efficacy remain unanswered. Prostate cancer also continues to be an area in which progress is needed despite major recent advancements. Numerous debates that include the value of PSA screening and appropriate roles for each of the numerous therapeutic modalities await resolution. For millions of patients who suffer from prostatitis, a major breakthrough is yet to come. Current treatment regimens for this important and prevalent clinical entity remain ineffective at best.

References

[1] Brooks JD. Anatomy of the lower urinary tract and male genitalia. In: Walsh PC, Retik AB, Vaughan ED, et al, editors. Campbell's urology. Philadelphia: Saunders; 2002. p. 41–80.

[2] Wendell-Smith C. Terminology of the prostate and related structures. Clin Anat 2000;13: 207–13.

[3] Laczko I, Hudson DL, Freeman A, et al. Comparison of the zones of the human prostate with the seminal vesicle: morphology, immunohistochemistry, and cell kinetics. Prostate 2005; 62:260–6.

[4] Partin AW, Rodriguez R. The molecular biology, endocrinology, and physiology of the prostate and seminal vesicles. In: Walsh PC, Retik AB, Vaughan ED, et al, editors. Campbell's urology. Philadelphia: Saunders; 2002. p. 1237–96.

[5] American Urological Association. AUA guideline on management of benign prostatic hyperplasia (2003). Chapter 1: diagnosis and treatment recommendations. J Urol 2003;170: 530–47.

[6] Thorpe A, Neal D. Benign prostatic hyperplasia. Lancet 2003;361:1359–67.

[7] McNeal J. Pathology of benign prostatic hyperplasia. Insight into etiology. Urol Clin North Am 1990;17:477–86.

[8] McNeal JE. Origin and evolution of benign prostatic enlargement. Invest Urol 1978;15: 340–5.

[9] Roehrborn CG, McConnell JD. Etiology, pathophysiology, epidemiology, and natrual history of benign prostatic hyperplasia. In: Walsh PC, Retik AB, Vaughan ED, et al, editors. Campbell's urology. Philadelphia: Saunders; 2002. p. 1297–336.

[10] Lepor H. The pathophysiology of lower urinary tract symptoms in the ageing male population. Br J Urol 1998;81(Suppl 1):29–33.

[11] Schwinn DA. Novel role for alpha1-adrenergic receptor subtypes in lower urinary tract symptoms. BJU Int 2000;86(Suppl 2):11–20 [discussion: 20–2].

[12] Lepor H, Gup DI, Baumann M, et al. Laboratory assessment of terazosin and alpha-1 blockade in prostatic hyperplasia. Urology 1988;32:21–6.

[13] Lepor H, Tang R, Meretyk S, et al. Alpha 1 adrenoceptor subtypes in the human prostate. J Urol 1993;149:640–2.

[14] Lee KL, Peehl DM. Molecular and cellular pathogenesis of benign prostatic hyperplasia. J Urol 2004;172:1784–91.

[15] Berry SJ, Coffey DS, Walsh PC, et al. The development of human benign prostatic hyperplasia with age. J Urol 1984;132:474–9.

[16] Homma Y, Kawabe K, Tsukamoto T, et al. Epidemiologic survey of lower urinary tract symptoms in Asia and Australia using the international prostate symptom score. Int J Urol 1997;4:40–6.

[17] Barry MJ, Fowler FJ Jr, O'Leary MP, et al. The American Urological Association symptom index for benign prostatic hyperplasia. The Measurement Committee of the American Urological Association. J Urol 1992;148:1549–57 [discussion: 1564].

[18] Roehrborn CG, Sech S, Montoya J, et al. Interexaminer reliability and validity of a three-dimensional model to assess prostate volume by digital rectal examination. Urology 2001;57:1087–92.

[19] Carvalhal GF, Smith DS, Mager DE, et al. Digital rectal examination for detecting prostate cancer at prostate specific antigen levels of 4 ng./ml. or less. J Urol 1999;161:835–9.

[20] Roehrborn CG, McConnell J, Bonilla J, et al. Serum prostate specific antigen is a strong predictor of future prostate growth in men with benign prostatic hyperplasia. PROSCAR long-term efficacy and safety study. J Urol 2000;163:13–20.

[21] Roehrborn CG, McConnell JD, Lieber M, et al. Serum prostate-specific antigen concentration is a powerful predictor of acute urinary retention and need for surgery in men with clinical benign prostatic hyperplasia. PLESS Study Group. Urology 1999;53:473–80.

[22] Roehrborn CG, Boyle P, Bergner D, et al. Serum prostate-specific antigen and prostate volume predict long-term changes in symptoms and flow rate: results of a four-year, randomized trial comparing finasteride versus placebo. PLESS Study Group. Urology 1999;54:662–9.

[23] Roehrborn CG, Malice M, Cook TJ, et al. Clinical predictors of spontaneous acute urinary retention in men with LUTS and clinical BPH: a comprehensive analysis of the pooled placebo groups of several large clinical trials. Urology 2001;58:210–6.

[24] Walmsley K, Gjertsen CK, Kaplan SA. Medical management of BPH—an update. In: Walsh PC, Retik AB, Vaughan ED, et al, editors. Campbell's urology updates. Philadelphia: Elsevier; 2004. p. 1–12.

[25] Flanigan RC, Reda DJ, Wasson JH, et al. 5-year outcome of surgical resection and watchful waiting for men with moderately symptomatic benign prostatic hyperplasia: a Department of Veterans Affairs cooperative study. J Urol 1998;160:12–6 [discussion: 16–7].

[26] Wasson JH, Reda DJ, Bruskewitz RC, et al. A comparison of transurethral surgery with watchful waiting for moderate symptoms of benign prostatic hyperplasia. The Veterans Affairs Cooperative Study Group on Transurethral Resection of the Prostate. N Engl J Med 1995;332:75–9.

[27] Temml C, Brossner C, Schatzl G, et al. The natural history of lower urinary tract symptoms over five years. Eur Urol 2003;43:374–80.

[28] Clifford GM, Farmer RD. Medical therapy for benign prostatic hyperplasia: a review of the literature. Eur Urol 2000;38:2–19.

[29] Barry MJ, Roehrborn CG. Benign prostatic hyperplasia. BMJ 2001;323:1042–6.

[30] Cabot AT. The question of castration for enlarged prostate. Ann Surg 1896;24:265–309.

[31] Chapple CR. Pharmacological therapy of benign prostatic hyperplasia/lower urinary tract symptoms: an overview for the practising clinician. BJU Int 2004;94:738–44.

[32] Bartsch G, Rittmaster RS, Klocker H. Dihydrotestosterone and the concept of 5alpha-reductase inhibition in human benign prostatic hyperplasia. Eur Urol 2000;37:367–80.

[33] Geller J. Effect of finasteride, a 5 alpha-reductase inhibitor on prostate tissue androgens and prostate-specific antigen. J Clin Endocrinol Metab 1990;71:1552–5.

[34] McConnell JD, Bruskewitz R, Walsh P, et al. The effect of finasteride on the risk of acute urinary retention and the need for surgical treatment among men with benign prostatic hyperplasia. Finasteride Long-Term Efficacy and Safety Study Group. N Engl J Med 1998;338:557–63.

[35] Roehrborn CG, Boyle P, Nickel JC, et al. Efficacy and safety of a dual inhibitor of 5-alpha-reductase types 1 and 2 (dutasteride) in men with benign prostatic hyperplasia. Urology 2002;60:434–41.

[36] Lepor H, Williford WO, Barry MJ, et al. The impact of medical therapy on bother due to symptoms, quality of life and global outcome, and factors predicting response. Veterans Affairs Cooperative Studies Benign Prostatic Hyperplasia Study Group. J Urol 1998;160:1358–67.

[37] Roehrborn CG, Bruskewitz R, Nickel GC, et al. Urinary retention in patients with BPH treated with finasteride or placebo over 4 years. Characterization of patients and ultimate outcomes. The PLESS Study Group. Eur Urol 2000;37:528–36.

[38] Gormley GJ, Stoner E, Bruskewitz RC, et al. The effect of finasteride in men with benign prostatic hyperplasia. The Finasteride Study Group. N Engl J Med 1992;327:1185–91.

[39] Roehrborn CG. Drug treatment for LUTS and BPH: new is not always better. Eur Urol 2005;49(1):5–7.

[40] Lepor H, Williford WO, Barry MJ, et al. The efficacy of terazosin, finasteride, or both in benign prostatic hyperplasia. Veterans Affairs Cooperative Studies Benign Prostatic Hyperplasia Study Group. N Engl J Med 1996;335:533–9.

[41] Debruyne FM, Jardin A, Colloi D, et al. Sustained-release alfuzosin, finasteride and the combination of both in the treatment of benign prostatic hyperplasia. European ALFIN Study Group. Eur Urol 1998;34:169–75.

[42] McConnell JD, Roehrborn CG, Bautista OM, et al. The long-term effect of doxazosin, finasteride, and combination therapy on the clinical progression of benign prostatic hyperplasia. N Engl J Med 2003;349:2387–98.

[43] Han M, Alfert HJ, Partin AW. Retropubic and suprapubic open prostatectomy. In: Walsh PC, Retik AB, Vaughan ED, et al, editors. Campbell's urology. Philadelphia: Saunders; 2002. p. 1423–33.

[44] Madersbacher S, Lackner J, Brossner C, et al. Re-operation, myocardial infarction and mortality after transurethral and open prostatectomy: a nation-wide, long-term analysis of 23,123 cases. Eur Urol 2005;47:499–504.

[45] Fitzpatrick JM, Mebust WK. Minimally invasive and endoscopic management of benign prostatic hyperplasia. In: Walsh PC, Retik AB, Vaughan ED, et al, editors. Campbell's urology. Philadelphia: Saunders; 2002. p. 1379–422.

[46] Mebust WK, Holtgrewe HL, Cockett AT, et al. Transurethral prostatectomy: immediate and postoperative complications. A cooperative study of 13 participating institutions evaluating 3,885 patients. J Urol 1989;141:243–7.

[47] McConnell JD, Barry MJ, Bruskewitz RC. Benign prostatic hyperplasia: diagnosis and treatment. Agency for Health Care Policy and Research. Clin Pract Guidel Quick Ref Guide Clin 1994;1–17.

[48] Tooher R, Sutherland P, Costello A, et al. A systematic review of holmium laser prostatectomy for benign prostatic hyperplasia. J Urol 2004; 171:1773–81.

[49] Peterson MD, Matlaga BR, Kim SC, et al. Holmium laser enucleation of the prostate for men with urinary retention. J Urol 2005;174: 998–1001 [discussion: 1001].

[50] Naspro R, Salonia A, Cestari A, et al. A critical analysis of laser prostatectomy in the management of benign prostatic hyperplasia. BJU Int 2005;96:736–9.

[51] Te AE. The development of laser prostatectomy. BJU Int 2004;93:262–5.

[52] Te AE, Malloy TR, Stein BS, et al. Photoselective vaporization of the prostate for the treatment of benign prostatic hyperplasia: 12-month results from the first United States multicenter prospective trial. J Urol 2004;172:1404–8.

[53] Reich O, Bachmann A, Siebels M, et al. High power (80 W) potassium-titanyl-phosphate laser vaporization of the prostate in 66 high risk patients. J Urol 2005;173:158–60.

[54] Malek RS, Kuntzman RS, Barrett DM. Photoselective potassium-titanyl-phosphate laser vaporization of the benign obstructive prostate: observations on long-term outcomes. J Urol 2005;174:1344–8.

[55] Tan AH, Gilling PJ, Kennett KM, et al. Long-term results of high-power holmium laser vaporization (ablation) of the prostate. BJU Int 2003;92:707–9.

[56] Hoffman RM, MacDonald R, Monga M, Wilt TJ. Transurethral microwave thermotherapy vs transurethral resection for treating benign prostatic hyperplasia: a systematic review. BJU Int 2004;94:1031–6.

[57] Naslund MJ. Transurethral needle ablation of the prostate. Urology 1997;50:167–72.

[58] Routh JC, Leibovich BC. Adenocarcinoma of the prostate: epidemiological trends, screening, diagnosis, and surgical management of localized disease. Mayo Clin Proc 2005;80: 899–907.

[59] Postma R, Schroder FH. Screening for prostate cancer. Eur J Cancer 2005;41:825–33.

[60] Feuer EJ, Merrill RM, Hankey BF. Cancer surveillance series: interpreting trends in prostate cancer—part II: cause of death misclassification and the recent rise and fall in prostate cancer mortality. J Natl Cancer Inst 1999;91:1025–32.

[61] Jemal A, Siegel R, Ward E, et al. Cancer statistics, 2006. CA: A Cancer Journal for Clinicians 2006;56:106–30.

[62] Polascik TJ, Oesterling JE, Partin AW. Prostate specific antigen: a decade of discovery—what we have learned and where we are going. J Urol 1999;162:293–306.

[63] Hankey BF, Feuer EJ, Clegg LX, et al. Cancer surveillance series: interpreting trends in prostate cancer—part I: evidence of the effects of screening in recent prostate cancer incidence, mortality, and survival rates. J Natl Cancer Inst 1999; 91:1017–24.

[64] Ross RK, Bernstein L, Lobo RA, et al. 5-alpha-reductase activity and risk of prostate cancer among Japanese and US white and black males. Lancet 1992;339:887–9.

[65] Bracarda S, de Cobelli O, Greco C, et al. Cancer of the prostate. Crit Rev Oncol Hematol 2005; 56:379–96.

[66] Carter BS, Steinberg GD, Beaty TH, et al. Familial risk factors for prostate cancer. Cancer Surv 1991;11:5–13.

[67] Carter BS, Bova GS, Beaty TH, et al. Hereditary prostate cancer: epidemiologic and clinical features. J Urol 1993;150:797–802.

[68] Spitz MR, Currier RD, Fueger JJ, et al. Familial patterns of prostate cancer: a case-control analysis. J Urol 1991;146:1305–7.

[69] Leitzmann MF, Stampfer MJ, Michaud DS, et al. Dietary intake of n-3 and n-6 fatty acids and the risk of prostate cancer. Am J Clin Nutr 2004;80: 204–16.

[70] Ganry O. Phytoestrogens and prostate cancer risk. Prev Med 2005;41:1–6.

[71] Shimizu H, Ross RK, Bernstein L, et al. Cancers of the prostate and breast among Japanese and white immigrants in Los Angeles County. Br J Cancer 1991;63:963–6.

[72] McCormack RT, Rittenhouse HG, Finlay JA, et al. Molecular forms of prostate-specific antigen and the human kallikrein gene family: a new era. Urology 1995;45:729–44.

[73] McGee RS, Herr JC. Human seminal vesicle-specific antigen is a substrate for prostate-specific antigen (or P-30). Biol Reprod 1988;39: 499–510.

[74] Stenman UH, Leinonen J, Alfthan H, et al. A complex between prostate-specific antigen and alpha 1-antichymotrypsin is the major form of prostate-specific antigen in serum of patients with prostatic cancer: assay of the complex improves clinical sensitivity for cancer. Cancer Res 1991;51:222–6.

[75] Stamey TA, Yang N, Hay AR, et al. Prostate-specific antigen as a serum marker for adenocarcinoma of the prostate. N Engl J Med 1987;317: 909–16.

[76] Catalona WJ, Richie JP, Ahmann FR, et al. Comparison of digital rectal examination and serum prostate specific antigen in the early detection of prostate cancer: results of a multicenter clinical trial of 6,630 men. J Urol 1994;151: 1283–90.

[77] Zhu H, Roehl KA, Antenor JA, et al. Biopsy of men with PSA level of 2.6 to 4.0 ng/mL associated with favorable pathologic features and PSA progression rate: a preliminary analysis. Urology 2005;66:547–51.

[78] D'Amico AV, Chen MH, Roehl KA, et al. Preoperative PSA velocity and the risk of death from prostate cancer after radical prostatectomy. N Engl J Med 2004;351:125–35.

[79] Shinohara K, Wheeler TM, Scardino PT. The appearance of prostate cancer on transrectal ultrasonography: correlation of imaging and pathological examinations. J Urol 1989;142: 76–82.

[80] Naughton CK, Miller DC, Mager DE, et al. A prospective randomized trial comparing 6 versus 12 prostate biopsy cores: impact on cancer detection. J Urol 2000;164:388–92.

[81] Rodriguez LV, Terris MK. Risks and complications of transrectal ultrasound guided prostate needle biopsy: a prospective study and review of the literature. J Urol 1998;160:2115–20.

[82] Pound CR, Partin AW, Epstein JI, et al. Prostate-specific antigen after anatomic radical retropubic prostatectomy. Patterns of recurrence and cancer control. Urol Clin North Am 1997;24:395–406.

[83] Cooner WH, Mosley BR, Rutherford CL Jr, et al. Prostate cancer detection in a clinical urological practice by ultrasonography, digital rectal examination and prostate specific antigen. J Urol 1990;143:1146–52 [discussion: 1152–4].

[84] Walsh PC, Jewett HJ. Radical surgery for prostatic cancer. Cancer 1980;45:1906–11.

[85] Rainwater LM, Morgan WR, Klee GG, et al. Prostate-specific antigen testing in untreated and treated prostatic adenocarcinoma. Mayo Clin Proc 1990;65:1118–26.

[86] Catalona WJ, Smith DS, Ornstein DK. Prostate cancer detection in men with serum PSA concentrations of 2.6 to 4.0 ng/mL and benign prostate examination. Enhancement of specificity with free PSA measurements. JAMA 1997;277:1452–5.

[87] Gleason DF. Classification of prostatic carcinomas. Cancer Chemother Rep 1966;50:125–8.

[88] D'Amico AV, Whittington R, Malkowicz SB, et al. A multivariate analysis of clinical and pathological factors that predict for prostate specific antigen failure after radical prostatectomy for prostate cancer. J Urol 1995;154:131–8.

[89] Partin AW, Kattan MW, Subong EN, et al. Combination of prostate-specific antigen, clinical stage, and Gleason score to predict pathological stage of localized prostate cancer. A multi-institutional update. JAMA 1997;277:1445–51.

[90] Terris MK, Klonecke AS, McDougall IR, et al. Utilization of bone scans in conjunction with prostate-specific antigen levels in the surveillance for recurrence of adenocarcinoma after radical prostatectomy. J Nucl Med 1991;32: 1713–7.

[91] Wolf JS Jr, Cher M, Dall'era M, et al. The use and accuracy of cross-sectional imaging and fine needle aspiration cytology for detection of pelvic lymph node metastases before radical prostatectomy. J Urol 1995;153:993–9.

[92] Mullerad M, Hricak H, Kuroiwa K, et al. Comparison of endorectal magnetic resonance imaging, guided prostate biopsy and digital rectal examination in the preoperative anatomical localization of prostate cancer. J Urol 2005;174: 2158–63.

[93] American Joint Committee on Cancer. Prostate. In: Greene, Frederick L, et al. AJCC cancer staging manual. New York: Springer-Verlag; 2002. p. 309.

[94] Carter HB, Walsh PC, Landis P, et al. Expectant management of nonpalpable prostate cancer with curative intent: preliminary results. J Urol 2002;167:1231–4.

[95] Allaf ME, Carter HB. The results of watchful waiting for prostate cancer. AUA Update Series 2005;24:1–7.

[96] Meraney AM, Haese A, Palisaar J, et al. Surgical management of prostate cancer: advances based on a rational approach to the data. Eur J Cancer 2005;41:888–907.

[97] Walsh PC, Donker PJ. Impotence following radical prostatectomy: insight into etiology and prevention. J Urol 1982;128:492–7.

[98] Rabbani F, Stapleton AM, Kattan MW, et al. Factors predicting recovery of erections after radical prostatectomy. J Urol 2000;164:1929–34.

[99] Trabulsi EJ, Guillonneau B. Laparoscopic radical prostatectomy. J Urol 2005;173:1072–9.

[100] Stolzenburg JU, Rabenalt R, Do M, et al. Endoscopic extraperitoneal radical prostatectomy: oncological and functional results after 700 procedures. J Urol 2005;174:1271–5 [discussion: 1275].

[101] Tewari A, El-Hakim A, Leung RA. Robotic prostatectomy: a pooled analysis of published literature. Expert Rev Anticancer Ther 2006;6:11–20.

[102] Woolsey J, Miller N, Theodorescu D. Permanent interstitial brachytherapy for prostate cancer: a current review. World J Urol 2003;21:209–19.

[103] Miller DC, Sandler H, Wei JT. Complications of permanent interstitial brachytherapy for carcinoma of the prostate. AUA Update Series 2004;23:9–15.

[104] Morris DE, Emami B, Mauch PM, et al. Evidence-based review of three-dimensional conformal radiotherapy for localized prostate cancer: an ASTRO outcomes initiative. Int J Radiat Oncol Biol Phys 2005;62:3–19.

[105] Hashine K, Numata K, Azuma K, et al. Long-term outcomes of 60 Gy conventional radiotherapy combined with androgen deprivation for localized or locally advanced prostate cancer. Jpn J Clin Oncol 2005;35:655–9.

[106] Mangar SA, Huddart RA, Parker CC, et al. Technological advances in radiotherapy for the treatment of localised prostate cancer. Eur J Cancer 2005;41:908–21.

[107] Horger DC, Clarke HS. Current status of cryosurgery in the treatment of prostate cancer. AUA Update Series 2004;23:145–51.

[108] Messing E. The timing of hormone therapy for men with asymptomatic advanced prostate cancer. Urol Oncol 2003;21:245–54.

[109] Damber JE. Endocrine therapy for prostate cancer. Acta Oncol 2005;44:605–9.

[110] Petrylak DP. Chemotherapy for androgen-independent prostate cancer. World J Urol 2005; 23:10–3.

[111] Schneider H, Ludwig M, Hossain HM, et al. The 2001 Giessen Cohort Study on patients with prostatitis syndrome—an evaluation of inflammatory status and search for microorganisms 10 years after a first analysis. Andrologia 2003; 35:258–62.

[112] Krieger JN, Nyberg L Jr, Nickel JC. NIH consensus definition and classification of prostatitis. JAMA 1999;282:236–7.

[113] Schneider H, Wilbrandt K, Ludwig M, et al. Prostate-related pain in patients with chronic prostatitis/chronic pelvic pain syndrome. BJU Int 2005;95:238–43.

[114] Krieger JN. Prostatitis revisited: new definitions, new approaches. Infect Dis Clin North Am 2003;17:395–409.

[115] Parsons CL, Rosenberg MT, Sassani P, et al. Quantifying symptoms in men with interstitial cystitis/prostatitis, and its correlation with potassium-sensitivity testing. BJU Int 2005;95: 86–90.

[116] Nickel JC. The three As of chronic prostatitis therapy: antibiotics, alpha-blockers and anti-inflammatories. What is the evidence? BJU Int 2004;94:1230–3.

[117] Alexander RB, Propert KJ, Schaeffer AJ, et al. Ciprofloxacin or tamsulosin in men with chronic prostatitis/chronic pelvic pain syndrome: a randomized, double-blind trial. Ann Intern Med 2004;141:581–9.

[118] Wyllie MG. Promise for prostatitis? BJU Int 2005;96:1137–8.

ELSEVIER
SAUNDERS

RADIOLOGIC
CLINICS
OF NORTH AMERICA

Radiol Clin N Am 44 (2006) 665–677

Inflammatory Disorders of the Prostate and the Distal Genital Tract

Jill E. Langer, MD[a],*, François Cornud, MD[b]

- Prostatitis
- Acute bacterial prostatitis
- Chronic bacterial prostatitis
- Prostate abscess
- Chronic nonbacterial prostatitis/chronic pelvic pain syndrome
- Asymptomatic prostatitis
- Granulomatous prostatitis
- MR imaging of prostatitis
- Evaluation of the ejaculatory ducts
- Invasive investigations for distal ejaculatory duct obstruction
- Partial ejaculatory duct stenoses
- Treatment of ejaculatory duct obstruction
- References

Inflammatory disease of the prostate and distal genital tract is emerging as major health problem because it estimated that up to 15% of adult men may be affected at some point in their lives [1,2]. A combination of thorough history taking, careful physical examination, and laboratory analysis can often lead the clinician to a correct diagnosis in affected men. Traditional imaging techniques such as retrograde urethrography provide only a limited assessment of the prostate, seminal vesicles, and ejaculatory system and have played a minor role in the evaluation of patients who have suspected inflammatory disease. Newer and continually improving imaging techniques such as high-resolution transrectal ultrasonography (TRUS) and MR imaging, however, offer the ability to view this portion of the urogenital tract with exquisite anatomic detail and often play a more crucial role in the evaluation of these patients.

Prostatitis

Prostatitis is thought to be the most common urologic disease in men younger than 50 years and the third most common in men older than 50 years [3]. Multiple population-based studies indicate that 2% to 10% of adult men have symptoms compatible with chronic prostatitis at any given time [1–5] and up to 14% to 16% may self-report a clinical history of prostatitis at some point in their lives [2]. Pathologically, prostatitis refers to inflammation of the prostate gland. Clinically, however, the diagnosis of "prostatitis" is used to refer to multiple disorders that cause pelvic pain and discomfort, ranging from acute bacterial infection to complex conditions that may not necessarily be caused by prostatic inflammation.

Traditionally, prostatitis has been divided into four subtypes based on the chronicity of symptoms, the presence of white blood cells in the prostatic

[a] Department of Radiology, Hospital of the University of Pennsylvania, University of Pennsylvania Medical Center, 3400 Spruce Street, Philadelphia, PA 19104, USA
[b] Hôpital Cochin, Service de Radiologie B, (Pr Chevrot), 27 rue du Fbg St Jacques, 75007 Paris, France
* Corresponding author.
E-mail address: jill.langer@uphs.upenn.edu (J.E. Langer).

0033-8389/06/$ – see front matter © 2006 Elsevier Inc. All rights reserved.
radiologic.theclinics.com

doi:10.1016/j.rcl.2006.07.004

fluid, and culture results [6–9]. These subtypes are acute bacterial prostatitis (ABP), chronic bacterial prostatitis, chronic nonbacterial prostatitis, and prostadynia. Because this etiology-based classification system did not always correlate with symptoms and therapeutic efficacy, particularly for the chronic forms of prostatitis, the International Prostatitis Collaborative Network of the National Institutes of Health (NIH) suggested a newer classification based mainly on symptomatology and examination of the prostatic expressate [5,7–9]. This classification merges chronic nonbacterial prostatitis and prostadynia into a single new category called chronic nonbacterial prostatitis/chronic pelvic pain syndrome (CNP/CPPS), which is further divided into inflammatory and noninflammatory subtypes based on the presence or absence of white blood cells in the prostatic secretions. In addition, the NIH proposed a new category of asymptomatic prostatitis (Table 1).

Acute bacterial prostatitis

ABP is a well-defined infectious disease that is relatively uncommon and can be considered a subtype of urinary tract infection. The prostate most likely becomes infected from reflux of urinary bacteria by way of the ejaculatory ducts (EDs) or from an ascending urethral infection [7,9,10]. The most common infectious agents include *Escherichia coli*, and other gram-negative rods, although a wide variety of pathogens has been reported [10,11]. Patients may present with fever, malaise, low back pain, dysuria, urgency, ejaculatory pain, and varying degrees of urinary obstruction depending on the severity and extent of urinary tract involvement. The prostate gland is typically tender, warm, swollen, and firm on digital rectal examination [7,9–11]. The diagnosis is made clinically and treated with antibiotics after isolating the bacteria by culturing the urine. Imaging is not necessary for the diagnosis but is useful to detect abscess formation in patients who are extremely ill or who fail to respond quickly to antibiotic therapy.

In uncomplicated ABP, imaging shows the hallmarks of acute inflammation: prostatic enlargement, surrounding edema, increased arterial flow, and venous engorgement [9,11,12]. On TRUS, the prostate changes from its typical ovoid or triangular appearance to a more rounded shape when viewed in the axial plane [9,13]. The overall echogenicity decreases secondary to edema, obscuring the echotexture differences between the peripheral zone and the central gland, with associated indistinctness of the capsule [13]. The gland may also appear heterogeneous, with small focal hypoechoic regions in the prostatic parenchyma—potential precursors to abscesses if not appropriately treated (Fig. 1) [9,10,13,14]. A hypoechoic halo in the periurethral area has also been described as a relatively specific sign of acute prostatitis, but this finding may be confused with the hypoechoic cylindric smooth muscle of the preprostatic sphincter, a normal structure that may be seen on TRUS [13]. Often marked increase in internal vascularity can be seen on color Doppler examination [12], particularly around the EDs and adjacent to the seminal vesicles. These changes are reversible following successful antibiotic therapy [9,12,13]. Although no truly specific sign has been identified, a sonographically normal gland usually excludes the diagnosis of ABP [13].

Chronic bacterial prostatitis

Patients who have chronic bacterial prostatitis experience recurrent clinical episodes of lower genitourinary tract infection caused by persistence of the same strain of pathogenic bacteria, usually *E coli* or another gram-negative rod [2]. Typically, chronic bacterial prostatitis occurs in older men, often with asymptomatic bacteruria. Many patients are asymptomatic between episodes of urinary tract infection and present with symptoms of dysuria, lower back or perineal pain, hematospermia, and occasional epididymo-orchitis. An infected prostate gland serves as the focus of these recurrent episodes of infection and can be diagnosed by demonstrating a high bacteria count and white bloods cells in the expressed prostatic secretions.

There are no distinct imaging features of chronic bacterial prostatitis when imaged between attacks

Table 1: Classification of prostatitis

Classic system	NIH	Categories
Acute bacterial prostatitis	I	Acute bacterial prostatitis
Chronic bacterial prostatitis	II	Chronic bacterial prostatitis
Chronic nonbacterial prostatitis	IIIa	Chronic nonbacterial prostatitis/Chronic pelvic pain syndrome with inflammatory cells present
Prostadynia	IIIb	Chronic nonbacterial prostatitis/Chronic pelvic pain syndrome without inflammatory cells present
	IV	Asymptomatic prostatitis

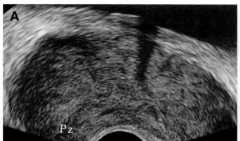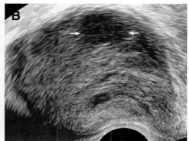

Fig. 1. Acute bacterial prostatitis. (*A*) Axial TRUS image in a 40-year-old patient who had acute prostatitis shows an enlarged and ovoid gland with overall decreased echogenicity. The differentiation between the peripheral zone (Pz), which is normally hyperechoic, and the central gland is difficult. (*B*) Sagittal TRUS image shows a focal hypoechoic region in the anterior central gland (*arrows*) representing a phlegmonous area of the prostate or early abscess formation.

[9,13]. The imaging findings may be similar to those of ABP during acute phases of inflammation, with glandular enlargement, hyperemia, and focal or global hypoechogenicity [9]. Over time, dystrophic calcification and fibrosis develops in the areas of recurrent inflammation. Although prostatic calcifications may be noted in many patients, calcifications in the apical peripheral zone (inferior to the verumontanum) are somewhat more specific for chronic bacterial prostatitis, reflecting the pathophysiology of reflux of infected urine into the prostatic parenchyma [9,13]. In general, the imaging features of chronic bacterial prostatitis are nonspecific and overlap with those of normals, patients who have benign prostatic hypertrophy, and chronic nonbacterial prostatitis as described later.

Prostate abscess

Prostate abscesses are relatively rare since the introduction of broad-spectrum antibiotics to treat urinary tract infections and the dramatic decrease in the incidence of gonococcal urethritis [10,15,16]. Intraprostatic abscesses, however, may be the sequelae of inappropriately or partially treated ABP or chronic bacterial prostatitis, or may develop de novo from hematogeneous seeding from a septic focus remote from the prostate. They develop in approximately 0.5% to 2.5% of patients hospitalized for prostatic inflammatory disease [9,10]. Risk factors include diabetes mellitus, chronic renal dialysis, hepatic cirrhosis, chronic urinary catheterization, and recent urethral manipulation [10,16]. A relatively new group of patients at risk includes those on immunosuppressive therapy or who have AIDS. In addition to bacterial infections, immunosuppressed patients may develop acute prostatitis and abscesses with atypical pathogens including viral and fungal infections [17,18].

Symptoms and clinical findings in patients who have a prostatic abscess are extremely variable and may be difficult to differentiate from other lower urinary tract inflammatory conditions. In one large series, fever was reported in only 60% of affected patients and perineal pain in only 20% [10]. Although digital rectal examination is painful in most patients, fluctuation and induration is not commonly noted [10,18]. A high degree of clinical suspicion is necessary to make the diagnosis because patients who have abscesses often require intervention.

TRUS is the most widely used technique for the diagnosis of a prostate abscess and is useful to guide percutaneous aspiration and drainage [15,18]. In general, abscesses over 1.5 cm require drainage, whereas smaller abscesses may be given a clinical trial of antibiotic therapy [15] TRUS-guided aspiration of the infected fluid in combination with intravenous antibiotics has a success rate of over 80% in curing the abscess [15,18]. Serial sonography may be used to document efficacy of therapy; surgical debridement may be necessary for treatment failures or extensive infection. TRUS demonstrates one or more irregularly shaped fluid collections, most typically with defined walls and less typically with poorly defined walls. The abscess often contains internal echoes and may be multiseptated [9–11,13,16,18]. Abscesses may involve any part of the gland but tend to be within the transitional zone [10]. Often a peripheral halo is seen with marked increased glandular and perilesional vascular flow. When the prostate is extensively involved, extension of the inflammatory process into one or both of the seminal vesicles is common. The affected seminal vesicle may appear enlarged (over 15 mm in diameter), with prominent luminal spaces containing complex fluid, or with larger complex abscess cavities (**Fig. 2**) [9,13].

CT is not typically necessary but is indicated in cases in which the abscess is suspected to have extended beyond the prostate or when there is concern for emphysematous prostatitis, a rare but

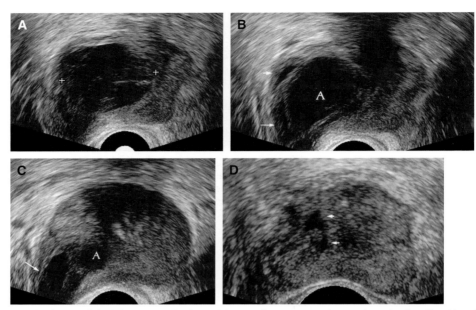

Fig. 2. Prostatic abscess. (A) Right parasagittal TRUS image shows a complex cystic cavity (outlined by electronic calipers) in the prostatic parenchyma, which proved to be a prostatic abscess in a 56-year-old man who had diabetes mellitus presenting with fever and perineal pain. (B) An axial view demonstrates subtle extension of the inflammation beyond the capsule into the adjacent periprostatic fat (*arrows*). A, abscess. (C) Axial TRUS image at the base of the prostate shows extension of the abscess (A) into the adjacent right seminal vesicle (*arrow*). (D) Axial TRUS image obtained 4 weeks after cystoscopic unroofing of the abscess demonstrates a minimal residual cavity (*arrows*).

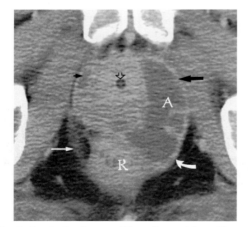

Fig. 3. Prostatic abscess. CT performed in a 62-year-old man for a fever of unknown origin shows a predominantly fluid-containing prostatic abscess (A), which extends to and bulges the prostate capsule (*large black arrowhead*). Posteriorly, the abscess extends beyond the prostate capsule (*curved white arrow*) and abuts the rectum (R). There are other heterogeneous regions of lower attenuation throughout the gland (*black arrowhead*) in addition to periprostatic inflammatory stranding (*white arrow*). Open arrow demonstrates a Foley catheter in the prostatic urethra.

important subtype of prostatitis that carries a higher mortality (Fig. 3) [19]. On CT, the inflamed prostate gland may appear enlarged, with adjacent stranding of the periprostatic fat [20,21]. Prostatic abscesses appear as multiple, well-demarcated fluid collections that have enhancing rims and may demonstrate internal septations (Fig. 4). CT imaging should include the kidneys and perineum to detect associated complications such as pyelonephritis and extension of the abscess beyond the prostate

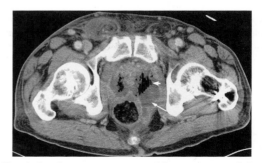

Fig. 4. Emphysematous prostatitis. A gas-containing prostatic abscess (*short arrow*) extending beyond the prostate into the perirectal fat (*long arrow*) developed following a *Klebsiella* urinary tract infection in a patient who underwent prolonged hospitalization for multiple medical problems including hepatic cirrhosis and type 2 diabetes mellitus.

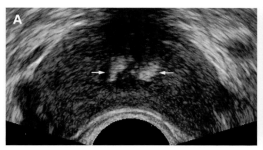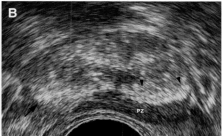

Fig. 5. Calcifications. (*A*) Axial TRUS image in a 45-year-old man who had a clinical history of recurrent bacterial prostatitis shows a small and diffusely hypoeochoic prostate with multiple periurethral calcifications (*arrows*) that likely occurred secondary to fibrosis from multiple bouts of infection. (*B*) Axial TRUS image in a different patient shows peripheral zone (PZ) calcifications (*large arrow*) and calcifications at the peripheral zone–central junction (*arrowheads*).

capsule into the adjacent tissues [20,21]. MR imaging performed in patients who have a prostatic abscess shows similar findings of one or typically multiple fluid collections with enhancing rims, replacing the prostatic parenchyma but preserving the internal architecture and prostatic capsule [17,22].

Chronic nonbacterial prostatitis/chronic pelvic pain syndrome

Although acute and chronic bacterial prostatitis represent the best understood prostate inflammatory disorders, they are the least common subtypes of prostatitis. More than 90% of symptomatic patients meet the criteria for the diagnosis of CNP/CPPS. These men have lower genitourinary pain with variable voiding and sexual dysfunction and without evidence of a bacterial infection or evidence of another etiology for their pain (such as urogenital cancer, urinary tract disease, active urethritis, urethral stricture, or neurologic disease affecting the bladder) [2]. Patients who have the inflammatory subtype of CNP/CPPS have leukocytes in the prostatic secretions, postprostatic message urine, or semen; the noninflammatory subtype patients do not. The etiology of CNP/CPPS is not clearly understood, and multiple disorders have likely been grouped together into this subcategory, including patients who have occult bacterial prostatitis, undiagnosed bladder pathology such as chronic cystitis, and neuromuscular syndromes.

The patient who has chronic prostatitis may prove to be very difficult to assess clinically and by imaging. Those affected have variable symptoms, waxing and waning over time. Pathologically, the affected prostate gland contains lymphocytes, plasma cells, and a few macrophages, ranging from minimal to extensive infiltration of the gland

[23,24]. Focal atrophy and microcalcifications are commonly noted.

The imaging findings reflect the variable clinical and histologic findings. TRUS findings include diffuse, focal, or multifocal hypoechoic changes in the peripheral zone. These hypoechoic lesions are most commonly multifocal patchy areas but may involve confluent areas of the peripheral zone (Fig. 5). A hypoechoic rim along the outer periphery of the prostate has also been described in patients who have chronic prostatitis [25] and shown to correlate with the degree of stromal fibrosis on histology. Rarely the inflammatory infiltration may be seen as a focal hypoechoic lesion, similar to prostate carcinoma; however, capsule deformity is uncommon and capsular interruption is absent.

Calcifications are a common finding in men who have chronic prostatitis; however, their clinical

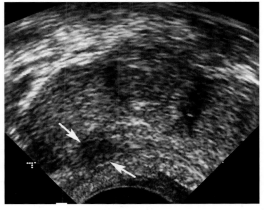

Fig. 6. Granulomatous prostatitis. Sagittal view of a 54-year-old man who had an elevated PSA shows a focal hypoechoic peripheral zone lesion (*arrows*). Biopsy showed changes of granulomatous prostatitis. The imaging features are indistinguishable from carcinoma and chronic prostatitis.

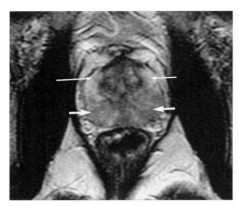

Fig. 7. MR imaging of chronic prostatitis. Coronal T2-weighted image of the prostate shows geographic regions of low signal (*thick arrows*) throughout most of the peripheral zone in a 28-year-old patient who had chronic prostatitis. A few regions of unaffected peripheral zone (*narrow arrows*) retain their normal high signal.

import is controversial. Endogenous calcifications, which derive from corporea amylacea, are made of lecithine and albuminous substance or come from the precipitation of anorganic substances present in the prostatic secretions [26]. Most of them are found in the transitional zone close to the surgical capsule or around the proximal prostatic

urethra (see Fig. 5) [9,24]. Conversely, exogenous calcifications are made of components of urine due to urine reflux through the prostatic ducts [26]. They are mainly found in the peripheral zone (see Fig. 5), which also often shows signs of chronic prostatitis. Small and multiple calcifications are asymptomatic and do not correspond to a prostatic inflammation [27]. Large and coarse calcifications are more often associated with clinical signs of chronic prostatitis [27]. In some cases, these large calcifications can also be found in the transition zone with concomitant inflammatory changes of the peripheral zone, suggesting that prostatitis can involve the peripheral and the transitional zones.

Abnormalities of one or both of the seminal vesicles, including dilation, elongation, and septal thickening may be seen in up to 20% of affected patients [25]. These findings, however, are nonspecific and overlap with patients who have benign prostatic hypertrophy and healthy control subjects [28,29]. Increased vascular flow may be present within the parenchyma, within the peripheral zone, surrounding the urethra, and surrounding the capsule [30]. Although the degree of inflammation correlates with the degree of increased vascularity, from a practical standpoint, color Doppler often adds little to the clinical diagnosis of chronic prostatitis or in differentiating the findings from prostate carcinoma [31–33].

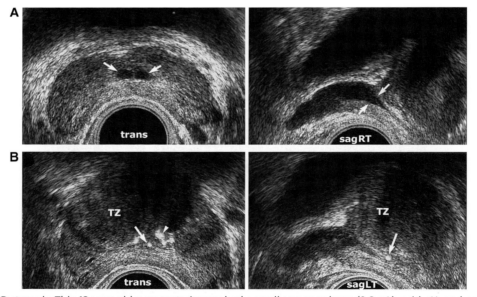

Fig. 8. ED stenosis. This 42-year-old azoospermic man had a small semen volume (0.8 mL), acid pH, and no semen fructose. (*A*) The transverse (trans) TRUS image on the left shows dilated EDs with a diameter greater than 2 mm (*arrows*). The right parasagittal (sagRT) TRUS image shows dilatation of the seminal vesicle (*arrows*). (*B*) The transverse (trans) TRUS image (*left panel*) shows the transitional zone (TZ) to be enlarged by changes of benign prostatic hypertrophy; corporea amylacea calcifications are present (*arrowheads*). A stone (*arrow*) is visible in the ejaculatory left duct. The left parasagittal (sagLT) TRUS image (*right panel*) also shows the stone (*arrow*) at the level of the verumontanum in the left ejaculatory duct.

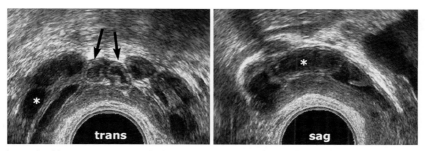

Fig. 9. Seminal vesicle dilation. Transverse (*left*) and sagittal (*right*) TRUS images show dilation of the ampullae of the vas deferens (*black arrows*) and the seminal vesicles (*asterisks*) in a 33-year-old azoospermic man who had a small semen volume (1.2 mL).

Asymptomatic prostatitis

This category is defined by the presence of inflammatory cells in prostatic secretions or during histologic review of the prostate in an otherwise asymptomatic patient. Common examples include the detection of prostatitis on needle biopsy specimens performed to exclude prostate carcinoma in patients who have elevated PSA levels or the detection of a large number of leukocytes in the seminal fluid of men being evaluated for infertility. The incidence of this type of prostatitis is unknown but was found to be as high as 32% when determined by seminal analysis of an asymptomatic population undergoing prostate cancer screening [34]. Inflammation is a frequent histologic finding on prostate biopsy specimens performed for elevated PSA, and higher PSA values have been noted in those who have more inflammation [35]. There is also evidence that antibiotic therapy and nonsteroidal medications can lower the PSA level in these patients [36].

Granulomatous prostatitis

Granulomatous prostatitis in an unusual benign inflammatory process that is not included in the NIH classification but is noted on histology in approximately 1.4% of resected prostate specimens [37]. Clinically, it may cause a focal lesion that can masquerade as prostatic carcinoma on digital rectal examination and TRUS and may cause transient elevation of PSA levels (Fig. 6). Prostatic enlargement and multifocal hypoechoic lesions may also

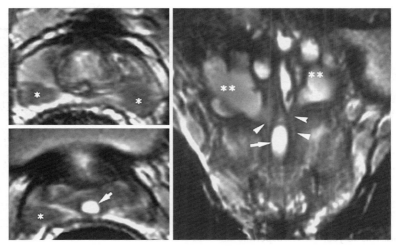

Fig. 10. Median cyst, chronic prostatitis, and ED distal stenosis in an azoospermic 34-year-old man who had a small ejaculate (1.1 mL). Endorectal MR images show a small median cyst (*arrows*) associated with several areas of low signal intensity within the peripheral zone, due to chronic prostatitis (*single asterisks*). On the coronal view (*right panel*), the seminal vesicles appear dilated (*double asterisks*). Caudal junctions of the vas deferens and the seminal vesicles are visible (*arrowheads*). EDO has been attributed to the combined effect of the cyst and prostatitis.

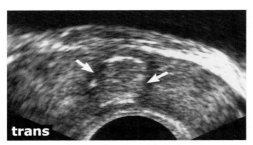

Fig. 11. Complicated median cyst in a 27-year-old man who had hematospermia, pollakiuria, and pelvic pain. Transverse TRUS image shows a median cyst (*arrows*) with calcified walls and hyperechoic contents due to intracystic infection or hemorrhage.

be noted [38]. Granulomatous prostatitis can be divided into the following four subtypes: idiopathic (nonspecific), infective, iatrogenic (postsurgical), and a miscellaneous category that includes malakoplakia and cases associated with systemic granulomatous diseases. Nonspecific granulomatous prostatitis is the most common type (over 60% of all cases) and is a self-limited benign condition that resolves without therapy, although it may cause considerable scarring of the gland. Infective granulomatous prostatitis can be caused by a variety of specific pathogens (most commonly *Mycobacterium tuberculosis*) or from intravesical bacillus Calmette-Guérin therapy for bladder cancer. Other infectious agents including *Treponema pallidum*, viruses, and various fungi have also been reported to be causes of granulomatous prostatitis. Iatrogenic granulomatous prostatitis is noted only in resected specimens of patients who previously underwent transurethral resection of the prostate and is thought to be a reactive phenomenon of the epithelium to previous trauma.

MR imaging of prostatitis

On MR imaging, lesions of chronic prostatitis and granulomatous prostatitis appear as low-signal intensity abnormalities in the peripheral zone that are indistinguishable from carcinoma [38]. Acute prostatitis may demonstrate patchy curvilinear regions of alternating high- and low-signal intensities or diffuse low to intermediate signal in the peripheral zone [39]. In ABP and chronic bacterial prostatitis, the central gland may show a ground glass-like homogeneous low-signal intensity, a finding initially reported in patients who had prostate carcinoma. Care must be taken, however, to avoid overdiagnosis because lower peripheral zone signal may be a normal finding in younger men [39]. Chronic prostatitis is seen most commonly as multifocal noncontour deforming areas that have low signal on T2-weighted images and is seen less commonly has a zonal distribution (Figs. 7, 10, 13) [40]. In the absence of invasion of the capsule or seminal vesicles, these lesions are indistinguishable from confined prostate carcinoma [39,40].

Evaluation of the ejaculatory ducts

The causes of ED obstruction (EDO) include midline or eccentric cysts, ED calcification or stones, and blockage by postoperative or postinfectious scar tissue [41,42]. Several causes are often associated in the same patient. Patients may present with pelvic pain, hematospermia, or infertility.

Complete distal stenosis of the EDs is detected in 5% of hypofertile men [41], of whom many have no known history of genital infection. Although the physical examination is often normal in affected patients, unilateral or bilateral epididymal enlargement can be found by palpation or scrotal sonography. The spermogram shows azoospermia, a small ejaculate volume (<1 to 1.5 mL), low pH, and no fructose. TRUS can detect signs of distal obstruction of the seminal tract. Dilatation of the EDs, seminal vesicles, or vas deferens can be obvious (Fig. 8). Dilatation of the vas deferens is less common, owing to the thick muscular wall of these structures (Fig. 9). Other common findings include unilateral

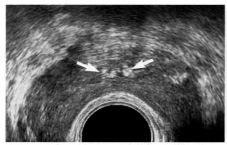
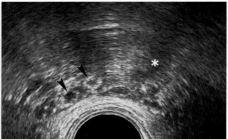

Fig. 12. Distal ED stenosis and retraction of the seminal vesicles. Transverse TRUS images in a 29-year-old man who had a small ejaculate (1 mL) and severe sperm abnormalities show multiple calcifications are visible around the ED (*left panel*) and markedly retracted seminal vesicles with hyperechoic calcified walls (*right panel, arrowheads*) and posterior acoustic shadowing (asterisk).

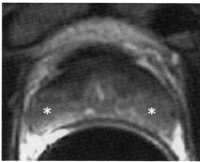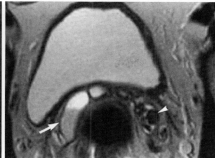

Fig. 13. Endorectal MR imaging. Axial T2-weighted images in a 34-year-old man who had a low semen volume and severe sperm abnormalities (sperm count <0.1 M, motility <5%, necrozoospermia >90%). Note the low signal intensity of the entire peripheral zone (*left panel, asterisks*) due to chronic prostatitis. There is dilatation of the right seminal vesicle due to obstruction (*right panel, arrow*) and retraction of the left seminal vesicle that contains dark signal voids corresponding to stones (*right panel, arrowhead*).

or bilateral lithiasis of the EDs or the vas deferens or seminal vesicles (see Fig. 8), which can be a cause or a consequence of ED stenosis. Small median or paramedian cysts may also be detected. If not themselves responsible for the obstruction, they are thought to be cofactors in distal stenosis (Fig. 10) [43]. In most cases, TRUS shows signs of chronic prostatitis in the peripheral zone, confirming the postinflammatory setting in which acquired distal stenoses occur. Patients who have hemospermia may have a median cyst complicated by intracystic infection or bleeding, which modifies the sonographic aspect of the cyst (Fig. 11). In some cases, inflammation can induce retraction of the seminal vesicles (Fig. 12). The obstruction is thus masked, and it becomes impossible to ascertain whether the low volume of ejaculate is due to seminal vesicle retraction, EDO, or both. MR imaging clearly shows the retraction of one or both seminal vesicles [44] when TRUS is inconclusive (Fig. 13). Patients must be screened for retraction of the seminal vesicles before contemplating antibiotic and anti-inflammatory therapy to increase semen fluidity.

Invasive investigations for distal ejaculatory duct obstruction

Surgical deferentography is being abandoned in favor of more accurate endorectal imaging. Distal endorectal imaging, however, cannot show whether distal EDO is associated with a more proximal obstruction, which is observed in 20% of cases [42]. TRUS-guided puncture aspiration of seminal vesicle fluid has been proposed to detect more proximal obstructions. In men who have distal EDO, sperm are detected in the seminal vesicles as they join the vas deferens to form the EDs before entering the prostatic tissue [45,46]. No sperm are found in the seminal vesicles 12 hours after ejaculation

in men who do not have EDO [47] because the spermatozoa are stored within the ampullae of the vas deferens. The absence of sperm in the seminal vesicles of a patient who has EDO suggests a more proximal obstruction or defective spermatogenesis. The suspected proximal obstruction can be located by transrectal vesiculography (Fig. 14) [48,49] with retrograde opacification of the vas deferens or by surgical deferentography.

Partial ejaculatory duct stenoses

Partial ED stenoses may be suspected in nonazoospermic patients who have sperm motility less

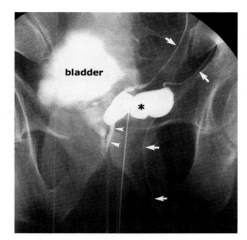

Fig. 14. TRUS-guided vesiculography. There is opacification of the left seminal vesicle (*asterisk*) of the normally patent left vas deferens (*arrows*) including the intrascrotal portion and of the left EDs (*arrowheads*) without obvious stenosis. Note the reflux into the bladder due to opening of the preprostatic sphincter induced by general anesthesia.

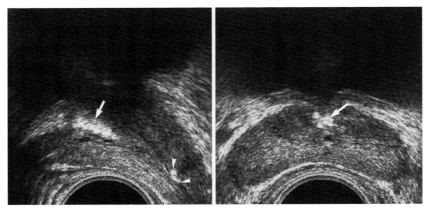

Fig. 15. Prostatic calcifications and hypofertility. Sagittal (*left panel*) and transverse (*right panel*) TRUS images show a large hyperechoic focus is located along the anterior aspect of the EDs (*arrows*), potentially inducing partial ED stenosis [57]. Calcifications located close to the verumontanum (*arrowheads*) are common in normofertile and hypofertile men.

than 30% [41], a reduced or normal sperm count [50], and an ejaculate volume close to the lower limit of normal (2 mL) [51] but are difficult to confirm. TRUS can show seminal vesicle enlargement (anterior-posterior diameter ≥ 15 mm) and roundish, anechoic areas in the seminal vesicles, reflecting stasis [52] or it can show calcifications around the EDs that are more frequently detected in hypofertile men [53]. MR imaging can detect early distension of the seminal vesicles (Fig. 15); however, Purohit and colleagues [41] suggested that more invasive or dynamic tests should be added to improve the accuracy of endorectal imaging. These investigators compared the accuracy of five TRUS signs of partial EDO (ED diameter >2 mm, anteroposterior axis of the seminal vesicles >15 mm, ED lithiasis, calcifications around the EDs, and median cysts) to that of

three invasive tests (TRUS-guided seminal vesicle puncture, vesiculography, and chromotubation). Chromotubation requires TRUS-guided injection of methylene blue into the seminal vesicles and visual cystoscopic verification of ED patency. Among 25 patients who had at least one TRUS sign of partial EDO, only 12 (48%) had EDO confirmed by one of the three invasive tests. The limitations of these invasive tests were underlined in the editorial comments at the end of the article, which pointed out that diagnosis of EDO based on vesiculography (no contrast material passing through the EDs) or chromotubation (no visible methylene blue) was questionable if sperm still passed through (most of the patients in the series were not azoospermic). It was concluded that the diagnosis of partial EDO remained investigational.

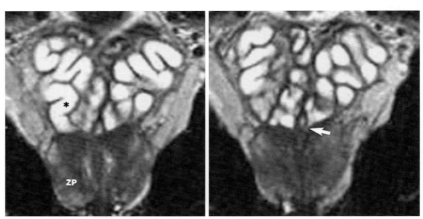

Fig. 16. Endorectal MR imaging and partial ED stenosis in a 34-year-old man who had a moderate reduction in semen volume (1.5 mL) and a reduced sperm count and motility. TRUS (not shown) showed enlarged but non-dilated seminal vesicles. The T2-weighted coronal views show moderately dilated seminal vesicles but distension at the level of the root of the right seminal vesicles (*right panel, arrow*), indicating distal ED obstruction. Note the areas of low signal intensity in the peripheral zone (ZP, *left panel*) due to chronic prostatitis.

Treatment of ejaculatory duct obstruction

Endoscopic resection is the most common treatment for EDO. It can involve resection of the verumontanum or of the roof of a median cyst. The best outcomes are obtained in men who have midline cysts treated by transurethral resection [54]. In patients who have EDO due to inflammatory stenosis, short stenoses are more likely than longer stenoses to respond favorably to resection [43]. The length of the stenosis can be accurately determined by endorectal imaging. Short stenoses involving only the lower portion of the EDs respond more favorably to resection than those involving the upper portion. Stenoses extending outside the prostate and involving the caudal junction of the vas deferens and the seminal vesicles are a contraindication to endoscopic resection (Fig. 16) [55]. Complications include chronic reflux of urine through the EDs, giving a watery ejaculate [51], and secondary fibrosis and reocclusion of the EDs, which occurs in approximately 4% of cases [50]. Candidates for

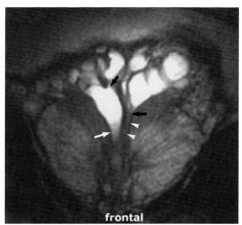

Fig. 17. Preoperative imaging in a man who had distal EDs. This 35-year-old patient was not azoospermic (sperm count 2 M/mL, motility 20%) but had a small ejaculate (1.1 mL). Both seminal vesicles were dilated on TRUS (not shown). The coronal view of a fast spin echo (FSE) T2-weighted MR imaging sequence confirmed the dilatation of both seminal vesicles. The caudal junction with the vas deferens is clearly outside the prostate tissue on the right (*right black arrow*) and the EDO is located at the lower third of the ED (*white arrow*). The junction is located much lower on the left side (*left black arrow*). The left ED is faintly visible (*arrowhead*), and it is not clear whether the junction is spared by the stenosis. Transurethral resection of the ED improved the sperm parameters (semen volume: 3.2 mL, sperm count 56 M/mL, motility 54%) sufficiently for cryopreservation. Two months later, sperm parameters returned to their values before resection, showing that the obstruction had recurred.

transurethral resection of the ED must therefore be selected with utmost care (Fig. 17).

Interventional radiology has been attempted in isolated cases. TRUS-guided puncture of a median cyst is a less aggressive procedure than transurethral resection of the ED [43,56]. Sperm parameters may improve dramatically in the short-term, but long-term patency rates (after 6 months) are not known. A single case of successful balloon dilatation of a unilateral ED stenosis based on a combined transrectal-transuretral approach has been reported [55], but long-term patency was not reported.

References

[1] Krieger JN. Classification, epidemiology and implications of chronic prostatitis in North America, Europe and Asia. Minerva Urol Nefrol 2004; 56(2):99–107.

[2] Nickel JC, Teichman JM, Gregoire M, et al. Prevalence, diagnosis, characterization, and treatment of prostatitis, interstitial cystitis, and epididymitis in outpatient urological practice: the Canadian PIE Study. Urology 2005;66(5):935–40.

[3] Collins MM, Stafford RS, O'Leary MP, et al. How common is prostatitis? A national survey of physician visits. J Urol 1998;159(4):1224–8.

[4] Moon TD, Hagen L, Heisey DM. Urinary symptomatology in younger men. Urology 1997; 50(5):700–3.

[5] Roberts RO, Lieber MM, Bostwick DG, et al. A review of clinical and pathological prostatitis syndromes. Urology 1997;49(6):809–21.

[6] Drach GW, Fair WR, Meares EM, et al. Classification of benign diseases associated with prostatic pain: prostatitis or prostatodynia? J Urol 1978; 120(2):266.

[7] Potter SR, Partin AW. Prostatitis syndromes and benign prostatic hyperplasia. Semin Roentgenol 1999;34(4):256–68.

[8] Nickel JC, Nyberg LM, Hennenfent M. Research guidelines for chronic prostatitis: consensus report from the first National Institutes of Health International Prostatitis Collaborative Network. Urology 1999;54(2):229–33.

[9] Wasserman NF. Prostatitis: clinical presentations and transrectal ultrasound findings. Semin Roentgenol 1999;34(4):325–37.

[10] Barozzi L, Pavlica P, Menchi I, et al. Prostatic abscess: diagnosis and treatment. AJR Am J Roentgenol 1998;170(3):753–7.

[11] Kravchick S, Cytron S, Agulansky L, et al. Acute prostatitis in middle-aged men: a prospective study. BJU Int 2004;93(1):93–6.

[12] Veneziano S, Pavlica P, Mannini D. Color Doppler ultrasonographic scanning in prostatitis: clinical correlation. Eur Urol 1995;28(1):6–9.

[13] Griffiths G, Clements R, Peeling W. Inflammatory disease and calculi. In: Resnick MI, editor. Prostate ultrasonography. Philadelphia: BC Decker; 1990. p. 123–52.

[14] Horcajada JP, Vilana R, Moreno-Martinez A, et al. Transrectal prostatic ultrasonography in acute bacterial prostatitis: findings and clinical implications. Scand J Infect Dis 2003;35(2): 114–20.

[15] Collado A, Palou J, Garcia-Penit J, et al. Ultrasound-guided needle aspiration in prostatic abscess. Urology 1999;53(3):548–52.

[16] Liu KH, Lee HC, Chuang YC, et al. Prostatic abscess in southern Taiwan: another invasive infection caused predominantly by *Klebsiella pneumoniae*. J Microbiol Immunol Infect 2003; 36(1):31–6.

[17] Fisher ME, Nisenbaum HL, Axel L, et al. Prostatic abscess due to *Aspergillus fumigatus*: TRUS and MR imaging findings. J Ultrasound Med 1998; 17(3):181–4.

[18] Lim JW, Ko YT, Lee DH, et al. Treatment of prostatic abscess: value of transrectal ultrasonographically guided needle aspiration. J Ultrasound Med 2000;19(9):609–17.

[19] Bae GB, Kim SW, Shin BC, et al. Emphysematous prostatic abscess due to Klebsiella pneumoniae: report of a case and review of the literature. J Korean Med Sci 2003;18(5):758–60.

[20] Thornhill BA, Morehouse HT, Coleman P, et al. Prostatic abscess: CT and sonographic findings. AJR Am J Roentgenol 1987;148(5): 899–900.

[21] Washecka R, Rumancik WM. Prostatic abscess evaluated by serial computed tomography. Urol Radiol 1985;7(1):54–6.

[22] Bertschinger K, Trinkler F, Reili I, et al. Sonographic and MR findings of an extensive, HIV-related prostatic abscess. J Magn Reson Imaging 1999;9(3):488–90.

[23] True LD, Berger RE, Rothman I, et al. Prostate histopathology and the chronic prostatitis/chronic pelvic pain syndrome: a prospective biopsy study. J Urol 1999;162(6):2014–8.

[24] Doble A, Carter SS. Ultrasonographic findings in prostatitis. Urol Clin North Am 1989;16(4): 763–72.

[25] Lee HJ, Choe GY, Seong CG, et al. Hypoechoic rim of chronically inflamed prostate, as seen at TRUS: histopathologic findings. Korean J Radiol 2001;2(3):159–63.

[26] Klimas R, Bennett B, Gardner WA Jr. Prostatic calculi: a review. Prostate 1985;7(1):91–6.

[27] Geramoutsos I, Gyftopoulos K, Perimenis P, et al. Clinical correlation of prostatic lithiasis with chronic pelvic pain syndromes in young adults. Eur Urol 2004;45(3):333–7 [discussion: 337–8].

[28] de la Rosette J, Karthaus H, Debruyne F. Ultrasonographic findings in patients with nonbacterial prostatitis. Urol Int 1992;48(3):323–6.

[29] Di Trapani D, Pavone C, Serretta V, et al. Chronic prostatitis and prostatodynia: ultrasonographic alterations of the prostate, bladder neck, seminal vesicles and periprostatic venous plexus. Eur Urol 1988;15(3–4):230–4.

[30] Cho IR, Keener TS, Nghiem HV, et al. Prostate blood flow characteristics in the chronic prostatitis/pelvic pain syndrome. J Urol 2000;163(4): 1130–3.

[31] Newman JS, Bree RL, Rubin JM. Prostate cancer: diagnosis with color Doppler sonography with histologic correlation of each biopsy site. Radiology 1995;195(1):86–90 [see comments].

[32] Rifkin MD, Sudakoff GS, Alexander AA. Prostate: techniques, results, and potential applications of color Doppler US scanning. Radiology 1993; 186(2):509–13.

[33] Patel U, Rickards D. The diagnostic value of colour Doppler flow in the peripheral zone of the prostate, with histological correlation. Br J Urol 1994;74(5):590–5.

[34] Carver BS, Bozeman CB, Williams BJ, et al. The prevalence of men with National Institutes of Health category IV prostatitis and association with serum prostate specific antigen. J Urol 2003;169(2):589–91.

[35] Schatteman PH, Hoekx L, Wyndaele JJ, et al. Inflammation in prostate biopsies of men without prostatic malignancy or clinical prostatitis: correlation with total serum PSA and PSA density. Eur Urol 2000;37(4):404–12.

[36] Bozeman CB, Carver BS, Eastham JA, et al. Treatment of chronic prostatitis lowers serum prostate specific antigen. J Urol 2002;167(4):1723–6.

[37] Mohan H, Bal A, Punia RP, et al. Granulomatous prostatitis—an infrequent diagnosis. Int J Urol 2005;12(5):474–8.

[38] Bude R, Bree RL, Adler RS, et al. Transrectal ultrasound appearance of granulomatous prostatitis. J Ultrasound Med 1990;9(12):677–80.

[39] Parsons RB, Fisher AM, Bar-Chama N, et al. MR imaging in male infertility. Radiographics 1997; 17(3):627–37.

[40] Ikonen S, Kivisaari L, Tervahartiala P, et al. Prostatic MR imaging. Accuracy in differentiating cancer from other prostatic disorders. Acta Radiol 2001;42(4):348–54.

[41] Purohit RS, Wu DS, Shinohara K, Turek PJ. A prospective comparison of 3 diagnostic methods to evaluate ejaculatory duct obstruction. J Urol 2004;171(1):232–5. [discussion: 235–6].

[42] Pryor J, Hendry W. Ejaculatory duct obstruction in subfertile males: analysis of 87 patients. Fertil Steril 1991;56:725–30.

[43] Cornud F, Belin X, Delafontaine D, et al. Imaging of obstructive azoospermia. Eur Radiol 1997;7(7):1079–85.

[44] Schnall MD, Pollack HM, Van Arsdalen K, et al. The seminal tract in patients with ejaculatory dysfunction: MR imaging with an endorectal surface coil. AJR Am J Roentgenol 1992;159(2): 337–41.

[45] Villers A, Terris MK, McNeal JE, et al. Ultrasound anatomy of the prostate: the normal gland and anatomical variations. J Urol 1990;143(4):732–8.

[46] Nguyen HT, Etzell J, Turek PJ. Normal human ejaculatory duct anatomy: a study of cadaveric

and surgical specimens. J Urol 1996;155(5): 1639–42.

[47] Jarow JP. Seminal vesicle aspiration of fertile men. J Urol 1996;156(3):1005–7.

[48] Riedenklau E, Buch JP, Jarow JP. Diagnosis of vasal obstruction with seminal vesiculography: an alternative to vasography in select patients. Fertil Steril 1995;64(6):1224–7.

[49] Jones TR, Zagoria RJ, Jarow JP. Transrectal US-guided seminal vesiculography. Radiology 1997; 205(1):276–8.

[50] Turek P, Magana J, Lipshultz L. Semen parameters before and after transurethral surgery for ejaculatory duct obstruction. J Urol 1996;155:1291–3.

[51] Goluboff E, Stifelman M, Fisch H. Ejaculatory duct obstruction in the infertile male. Urology 1995;45:925–31.

[52] Colpi GM, Negri L, Nappi RE, et al. Is transrectal ultrasonography a reliable diagnostic approach in ejaculatory duct sub-obstruction? Hum Reprod 1997;12(10):2186–91.

[53] Poore RE, Jarow JP. Distribution of intraprostatic hyperchoic lesions in infertile men. Urology 1995;45(3):467–9.

[54] Paick JS. Transurethral resection of the ejaculatory duct. Int J Urol 2000;7(Suppl):S42–7.

[55] Jarow JP, Zagoria RJ. Antegrade ejaculatory duct recanalization and dilation. Urology 1995; 46(5):743–6.

[56] Migliari R, Scarpa RM, Campus G. Percutaneous drainage of utricular cyst under ultrasound guidance. Br J Urol 1988;62:385–6.

[57] Jarow JP. Transrectal ultrasonography of infertile men. Fertil Steril 1993;60(6):1035–9.

ELSEVIER
SAUNDERS

RADIOLOGIC
CLINICS
OF NORTH AMERICA

Radiol Clin N Am 44 (2006) 679–687

Transrectal Sonography in Prostate Evaluation

Judd Boczko, MD[a], Edward Messing, MD[a], Vikram Dogra, MD[b],*

- Anatomy and embryology
- Sonographic anatomy
- Benign prostatic hyperplasia
- Prostate cancer
- Screening protocols
- Prostate-specific antigen
- Prostate biopsy

Indication for prostate biopsy
Patient preparation
Anesthesia
Technique
Repeat biopsy
Contraindications/complications
- Summary
- References

Transrectal ultrasonography (TRUS) was first introduced by Watanabe and colleagues [1–3] and later refined in technique and application by many investigators. The lack of ionizing radiation to the patient or examiner, the availability of lightweight handheld probes, the relative ease of mastering the basics of the transrectal sonographic prostate biopsy technique, and the ability to image the gland with precise volumetric measurements have contributed to the widespread clinical application of TRUS, particularly because there is an exponential rise in the number of men undergoing prostate biopsy after prostate-specific antigen (PSA) screening. Although TRUS is useful in imaging the prostate and is accurate in measuring prostate size, diagnostic accuracy in pinpointing cancerous areas is still lacking. In addition, there is no consensus regarding the optimal number of biopsy cores or a standardized patient preparation protocol. This article reviews the indications and principles of TRUS of the prostate, the technique of TRUS, and controversies pertaining to prostate core biopsy.

Anatomy and embryology

The prostate's embryologic origin is the terminal end of the hindgut, termed the *cloaca* (Latin, meaning sewer). The cloaca is divided by the urorectal septum at about 28 days of gestation. It eventually develops separately into the rectum and urogenital sinus, which are evident by 44 days of gestation [4]. The prostate first appears and starts its development from the urogenital sinus during the third month of fetal growth, and the development is primarily influenced by dihydrotestosterone, not testosterone. Dihydrotestosterone is produced from testosterone through the enzyme 5-α reductase, located within the urogenital sinus [5].

[a] Department of Urology, University of Rochester Medical Center, 601 Elmwood Ave, Rochester, NY 14642, USA
[b] University of Rochester School of Medicine, Department of Imaging Sciences, University of Rochester Medical Center, 601 Elmwood Ave, Box 648, Rochester, NY 14642, USA
* Corresponding author.
E-mail address: vikram_dogra@urmc.rochester.edu (V. Dogra).

0033-8389/06/$ – see front matter © 2006 Elsevier Inc. All rights reserved.
radiologic.theclinics.com

doi:10.1016/j.rcl.2006.07.001

The normal adult prostate weighs 18 g; measures 3 cm in length, 4 cm in width, and 2 cm in depth; and is traversed by the prostatic urethra. The prostate has been described as having a walnut shape. It has anterior, posterior, and lateral surfaces, with a narrow apex inferiorly and a broad base superiorly. It is enclosed by a fibromuscular stroma; however, no true capsule surrounds the apex of the prostate, which is continuous with the striated urethral sphincter. No true capsule separates the base of the prostate from the bladder. The arterial supply to the prostate is from the inferior vesical artery. Lymphatic drainage is primarily to the obturator and internal iliac nodes; however, a small portion can drain to the presacral and external iliac nodes. The cavernosal nerves run posterolaterally to the prostate within the lateral prostatic fascia [5].

Sonographic anatomy

The prostate is composed of approximately 70% glandular elements and 30% fibromuscular stroma. The glandular elements of the prostate are divided into discrete zones that can be clearly seen by TRUS (Fig. 1). The ducts of the transition zone arise at the angle dividing the preprostatic and prostatic urethra and go along its lateral and posterior sides. The transition zone contains 5% to 10% of the normal glandular tissue. A band of fibromuscular tissue separates the transition zone from the other glandular elements of the prostate. Although the transition zone is the usual origin of benign prostatic

hyperplasia (BPH), it can account for approximately 20% of prostate adenocarcinoma [5]. The ducts of the central zone surround the openings of the ejaculatory ducts. The central zone ducts compose about 25% of the normal glandular tissue and expand in a cone shape around the ejaculatory ducts to the base of the bladder. Only 1% to 5% of prostate cancers originate in this zone. The peripheral zone constitutes approximately 70% of the normal glandular tissue and covers the posterior and lateral aspects of the gland. Seventy percent of prostate adenocarcinomas originate in this zone, the zone most affected by chronic prostatitis [5]. The nonglandular fibromuscular stroma, which runs anteriorly from the bladder neck to the striated urinary sphincter, is rarely a site for the origin of prostate cancer. As opposed to this zonal anatomy, clinical classification of the prostate divides the gland into two palpable lateral lobes separated by a central sulcus and one nonpalpable median lobe that may project into the bladder in older men [5,6].

Benign prostatic hyperplasia

The prostate gland is a source of two common diseases that occur in men as they age: BPH and prostate cancer. BPH, the most common benign neoplasm in American men, is a chronic condition associated with progressive lower urinary tract symptoms (LUTS) that affects almost three out of four men during the seventh decade of life [7]. BPH is a result of

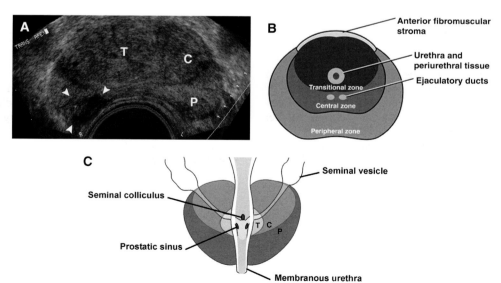

Fig. 1. Prostate anatomy. (*A*) Transrectal axial sonogram of the prostate gland. Arrowheads in the peripheral zone depict a hypoechoic lesion, confirmed to be prostate cancer. C, central zone; P, peripheral zone; T, transitional zone. (*B* and *C*) Diagrammatic representation of prostate gland zonal anatomy in axial (*B*) and coronal (*C*) planes.

the growth of epithelial and stromal cells. It begins in the transition zone and usually expands to compress its surrounding fibromuscular band into a pseudocapsule [8]. Clinically, patients progressively develop LUTS. These symptoms are variable and include nocturia, hesitancy, urgency, frequency, and incomplete voiding [7]. Numerous conditions can produce LUTS, so BPH cannot be solely diagnosed by such symptoms. In addition, prostate size alone correlates poorly with LUTS [9]. Because of this poor correlation, ultrasound is not a tool used in the diagnosis of BPH. Instead, it is used as a noninvasive method to determine postvoid residual volume in a patient [5]. Studies indicate that residual urine normally ranges from 0.09 to 2.24 mL [5]. Transabdominal ultrasound can help assess prostate size, intravesical filling defects, bladder diverticula, and thickness of the bladder wall [4]. For more accurate measurement of prostate size, TRUS should be performed with at least a 7.5-MHz transducer. Early degrees of BPH increase the anteroposterior dimension of the prostate due to transitional zone enlargement. The peripheral zones are normal in the early stages of BPH; however, as the prostate gland gets larger, the peripheral zones are compressed by the transitional zone and become more echogenic. The bladder base elevates and eventually, if the prostate gets large enough, the transrectal probe will not be able to be inserted deep enough to image the base of the prostate [5].

It is a combination of criteria including symptom severity, increased prostate size, abnormal uroflow results, and increased postvoid urine residue that aids in the diagnosis of BPH [5,10]. Watchful waiting is an acceptable approach in men who have mild symptoms of BPH [11]. In men suffering from LUTS, medical treatment of BPH with the use of α-blockers and 5-α reductase inhibitors is considered the first line of therapy [7]: α-blockers are the initial choice of medical therapy and act on the dynamic component of bladder outlet obstruction and relax the prostatic smooth muscle; 5-α reductase inhibitors act on the static component of bladder outlet obstruction and reduce prostate size by inhibiting the conversion of testosterone to dihydrotestosterone [12]. In the Medical Therapy of Prostatic Symptoms clinical trial, the combination of the two classes of medications was found useful in men who had larger prostates, specifically those greater than 40 g [13]. When medical therapy is no longer effective or cannot be tolerated, surgical therapy is the next option. Over the last several years, new minimally invasive surgical techniques have been developed to treat BPH, including transurethral microwave therapy, indigo laser therapy, and laser enucleation of the prostate [7,11]. The "gold standard" of BPH surgery, however, remains the transurethral resection of the prostate [14,15]. Regardless of what therapy is used, BPH is a highly prevalent, significant chronic condition that requires long-term care and evaluation.

Prostate cancer

Prostate cancer is the most prevalent newly diagnosed noncutaneous malignancy in men, second only to lung cancer in causing cancer-related deaths [16]. Screening with PSA blood tests and a digital examination has resulted in this earlier detection of the disease, allowing more patients to get primary curative treatment for their cancer.

Screening protocols

Downward stage and risk migration during the era of PSA screening is a well-established phenomenon. Most cases are now diagnosed at clinical stage T1c (nonpalpable; diagnosed by PSA) [17]. The percentage of patients presenting with locally advanced disease (T3-4; cancer has spread beyond the prostate) fell from 19.2% in 1988 to 4.4% in 1998; rates of metastatic disease at diagnosis also have decreased from 14.1% in 1988 to 3.3% in 1998 [18]. These statistics are most likely due to PSA screening and the adoption of extended-template prostate biopsy techniques [19,20]. It is therefore imperative to understand screening protocols and biopsy techniques.

As a screening tool, PSA is the best single test for the detection of early prostate cancer; however, the combination of PSA and a rectal examination is required because as many as 20% of prostate cancers with aggressive pathologic features are found in men who have a PSA level less than 4.0 ng/mL [21]. On digital examination, evaluation is performed for any obvious nodules, firmness, induration, or asymmetry within the prostate. The digital rectal examination is performed by a sweeping motion from the right to the left side, with the finger on the posterior aspect of the prostate, starting at the base, and then continuing to the mid and apex of the gland.

Prostate-specific antigen

PSA was first identified in the 1970s [22]. It is a serine protease that is expressed in high concentrations in seminal fluid where it is mostly unbound and plays a role in the liquefaction of seminal coagulum [23]. It is found in low concentrations in the serum, where it circulates in bound and unbound forms. Most PSA is in bound form and is covalently bonded to serine protease inhibitors such as alpha$_1$-antichymotrypsin and alpha$_2$-macroglobulin [24]. In the absence of prostate cancer, serum PSA levels can vary depending on age, race, and prostate volume. In general, a "normal" PSA value is below 4 ng/mL. This PSA threshold, however, can be adjusted to affect sensitivity and specificity. In reports from a large prostate cancer prevention trial in which all participants were asked to undergo an end-of-study biopsy regardless of PSA and digital rectal examination findings, no lower limit of PSA was found below which prostate cancer was extremely rare (ie, for PSA levels <1.0 ng/mL, over 7% had prostate cancer on six core template biopsies) [25]. Because of these factors, other means of using PSA as a screening tool have been explored. PSA velocity and age-adjusted PSA levels are used to lower the threshold level and increase sensitivity. PSA velocity measures the rate of change in PSA over an elapsed period of time. An abnormal PSA velocity is an increase of greater than 0.75 ng/mL per year [26]. This sort of elevation over a 1-year period is not typical of BPH and indicates malignant or inflammatory changes in the prostate [26]. Lowering the threshold to account for testing in a younger man (such as 2.5 ng/mL in men younger than 50 years and 3.5 ng/mL in men younger than 60 years) is another way to increase the detection rate of prostate cancer.

In contrast, evaluating PSA density is a method to increase the specificity of the PSA test. The PSA density is the quotient of the PSA level and the ultrasound-determined prostate volume. This calculation allows prostate volume to account for an elevated PSA as opposed to just assuming it is related to cancer. A PSA density of greater than 0.15 has been proposed as a threshold for recommending prostate biopsy [27]. Another method to increase specificity without a loss of sensitivity is to measure the ratio of free, unbound PSA to total PSA. The proportion of free PSA is lower in patients who have prostate cancer [28]. This ratio is especially useful in men who have total PSA values between 4 and 10 ng/mL. This range is often termed a "gray zone," depending on a patient's age and prostate volume. It is in this PSA range that performing a biopsy is most often questioned. In a large prospective study, Catalona and colleagues [29] found that a 25% free PSA cutoff would achieve a sensitivity of 95% and a specificity of 20%. More recently, a newer test has been designed to calculate pro-PSA, a precursor form of the PSA serum marker. The ratio of pro-PSA to free PSA improves the specificity of prostate cancer screening [30]. In one study, a percentage pro-PSA (ratio of pro-PSA to free PSA) cutoff of 1.8% was found to be superior to percentage free PSA in detecting prostate cancer in the PSA range between 2 and 10 ng/mL.

In addition, percentage pro-PSA was significantly increased in high-grade disease and had an increased selectivity for detecting more aggressive cancers [30].

Prostate biopsy

Indication for prostate biopsy

A prostate biopsy is generally recommended when a patient's PSA level is elevated or an abnormal digital rectal examination is noted (Box 1). Relative indications of biopsy include performing the biopsy before surgical treatment of BPH and before the use of salvage local therapy to diagnose (and stage) recurrence of prostate cancer in patients suspected of failing radiation therapy. A common exception to immediately recommending a biopsy for these indications is when an elevation of PSA occurs with a recent case of suspected prostatitis. In this scenario, a physician should prescribe a 3-week course of antibiotics and repeat the PSA test 2 to 3 months later. This practice allows enough time for prostatic tissue to return to its baseline state. When rechecking the PSA, the threshold for performing a biopsy should be very low, especially for a patient who has never had a biopsy.

Patient preparation

In preparation for a biopsy, patients must stop taking anticoagulants such as aspirin and warfarin sodium until their effects are minimized. Recent studies suggest that a biopsy can be performed in men taking aspirin without an increased risk of bleeding [31]. Although antibiotic prophylaxis is routinely advocated, no national guideline protocol has been developed. The authors' initial recommendation is for a patient to take a fluoroquinolone the morning of the biopsy until 2 days afterward. Patients who have a history of valvular heart disease, artificial joints, or vascular prostheses may need additional antibiotics. The American Heart

---

Box 1:   Indications for prostate biopsy

Absolute
- Elevated PSA
- PSA velocity >0.75 ng/mL per year
- Abnormal digital rectal examination

Relative
- Free PSA <20% when total PSA is in gray zone
- Ratio of pro-PSA to free PSA >1.8%
- Prior to surgery for BPH
- Prior to the use of salvage local therapy to diagnose and stage recurrence of prostate cancer after failed radiation therapy

Association recommends the administration of 2 g of ampicillin intramuscularly/intravenously at least 30 minutes before biopsy in moderate-risk patients. Those who are allergic to penicillin may substitute 1 g of vancomycin 1 to 2 hours before the procedure and complete it 30 minutes beforehand. High-risk patients need to add 120 mg of gentamicin intramuscularly 30 minutes before the biopsy and receive a second dose of ampicillin 6 hours later [32]. The use of prebiopsy enemas is controversial. Those who recommend it believe it improves ultrasound imaging and reduces the risk of bacterial infection from the biopsy [33]. Some studies have documented no benefit from the use of prebiopsy enemas [34,35]. In fact, an enema might increase the amount of feces in the lower rectum, which is normally empty except during defecation [36].

Ultrasound imaging is now routinely used during a biopsy. TRUS has two purposes. The first is to give the physician a visual aid in performing a systematic biopsy of the entire prostate. The second is to estimate prostate volume. Knowledge of prostate volume can be helpful when recommending treatment to a patient diagnosed with prostate cancer. If a patient is not diagnosed with cancer, then prostate volume assessment might help direct patient therapy for obstructive voiding symptoms. If ultrasound reveals a hypoechoic lesion within the prostate, it is more likely to harbor malignancy than normal tissue (Fig. 2). Ultrasound, however, is not reliable enough to use solely as a template for biopsy [37]. Other abnormalities that can cause hypoechoic changes include atrophy, prostatitis, and prostatic intraepithelial neoplasia. Ultrasound-distinct lesions that reveal cancer usually correlate with an abnormal digital rectal examination in that area [37]. If ultrasound reveals a lesion, then a biopsy must be performed separately or be incorporated into the systematic biopsy that is described later.

With the knowledge that prostate cancer has neovascularity [38], some reports have associated an increased vascularity in hypoechoic gray-scale lesions with an increased likelihood of cancer in the prostate [39,40]; however, when vascular areas were formally evaluated using two quantitative methods of vascularity assessment for the prostate (color and power Doppler imaging), the vascular areas did not distinguish cancer types and hypervascular hypoechoic areas did not increase the likelihood of cancer [41]. Recent development of the use of contrast-enhanced power Doppler ultrasonography has shown promise. Conventional color Doppler ultrasound's inability to help increase the detection rate of cancer might be attributed to the limited spatial resolution of ultrasound equipment combined with the prostatic area having small vessels with slow flow [42]. Intravascular contrast agents, however, can enhance the back-scattered echo from blood flow in these vessels and possibly increase the sensitivity of detecting cancer [43]. There has been some controversy over the helpfulness of contrast-enhanced Doppler ultrasound. In a study that looked at the vascular morphologic appearance of nodules and the role of sonocontrast agents, contrast-enhanced power Doppler sonography did not significantly aid in the diagnosis of prostate cancer [44]. In another study that evaluated the impact of using contrast-enhanced color Doppler targeted and systematic biopsy, however, the combined approach allowed for better detection of prostate cancer [42]. Further studies need to be performed to evaluate whether contrast-enhanced color flow Doppler significantly increases the detection rate of prostate cancer.

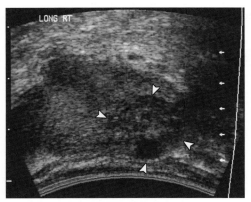

Fig. 2. Prostate cancer. Sagittal sonogram of the prostate gland reveals prostatic carcinoma as a hypoechoic area within the peripheral zone (*arrowheads*).

Anesthesia

In 1996, Nash and colleagues [45] were the first to describe the use of local anesthesia as a periprostatic block when performing a biopsy. Although initially slow to be accepted by urologists, it is now standard practice to administer anesthesia at the beginning of a biopsy, before the prostate volume is calculated. The method at the authors' institution is the following:

1. The patient is placed in a left lateral decubitus position with knees flexed.
2. A lubricated ultrasound probe is gently inserted into the patient.
3. The probe is set for sagittal and longitudinal views in a dual-screen image.
4. A 22-gauge spinal needle is inserted through the biopsy guide channel under ultrasound

guidance and directed toward the junction between the seminal vesicles and the prostate.

5. Five milliliters of plain lidocaine is injected into each side. A wheal between the seminal vesicles and prostate should appear.

6. The needle is removed in the same direction of insertion to decrease bleeding risks.

Technique

Over the years, there has been ongoing controversy as to how many cores should be obtained for an optimal prostate biopsy. In 1989, Hodge and colleagues [46] reported increased cancer detection rates using sextant biopsies rather than solely taking biopsies of palpable lesions and abnormal radiologic areas. A sextant biopsy involves obtaining 6 cores in the parasagittal line, halfway between the lateral border and midline of the prostate on each side of the prostate from the base, mid, and apex of the gland (Figs. 3 and 4). Using the sextant biopsy technique, cancer detection rates for PSA levels between 4 and 10 ng/mL were between 20% and 30%. When the PSA level was greater than 10 ng/mL, the yield increased to 50% to 70%. Keetch and colleagues [47], however, later showed that immediate repetition of sextant biopsy increased the detection rate by another 20%, thereby revealing a large sampling error inherent in the sextant biopsy. Using computer simulations of prostatectomy specimens that compared the location of the cancer in the gland to the direction of a biopsy needle, two studies concluded that a 10-core biopsy (peripheral, base, mid, apex, and two midline sagittal) would be optimal [48,49]. Because the anesthetic block was becoming more accepted and used and the patients were becoming less uncomfortable,

restrictions on the number of cores taken were erased. The advantage of a more extensive biopsy (>10 cores) was described in 2000 by Ravery and colleagues [50] who reported increased yields of 21.7% in men who had PSA levels less than 10 ng/mL and 12.7% in men who had PSA levels greater than 10 ng/mL compared with the sextant biopsy. Subsequent studies confirmed a greater detection rate using 12 to 14 cores [51–53]. A few centers currently have gone so far as to perform saturation biopsies (20–24 cores) [54]. It has not been definitively proven that sampling more than 10 cores detects significantly more cancers than the 10-core technique. The protocol used in the authors' institution is detailed in Box 2.

Repeat biopsy

Even with newer strategies, many patients undergo a negative biopsy but continue to have abnormal biochemical parameters. When such a patient has a persistently elevated PSA, an abnormal digital rectal examination, or a prostatic intraepithelial neoplasia in the initial biopsy, a repeat biopsy is recommended. When performing a repeat biopsy, attention should be directed to areas that were not sampled in the initial biopsy, including the anterior horn of the peripheral zone, lateral areas, and the transitional zone. In addition, an attempt should be made to take as many cores as the patient tolerates (up to 24 cores) to avoid the need for biopsies in the near future.

Contraindications/complications

Potential complications of the transrectal prostate biopsy may include rectal or urethral bleeding if all aspirin products are not stopped 7 to 10 days before biopsy if and warfarin sodium is not stopped 3 to 5 days before biopsy. If rectal

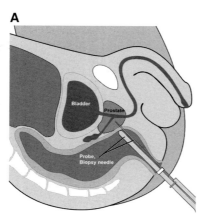
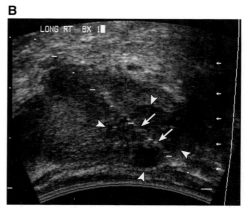

Fig. 3. (A) Diagrammatic representation of the technique of TRUS-guided prostate biopsy. (B) Sagittal sonogram demonstrates a biopsy needle (*arrows*) coursing through a hypoechoic area within the peripheral zone (*arrowheads*). It was confirmed to be prostatic adenocarcinoma.

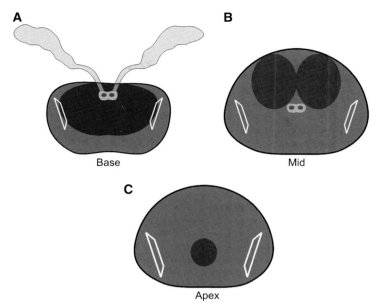

A

Base

B

Mid

C

Apex

Fig. 4. (*A–C*) Sextant biopsy. Diagrammatic representation of sextant biopsy from base (*A*) to mid (*B*) to apex (*C*) of the prostate gland. Trapezoid represents the biopsy needle.

bleeding occurs at the time of biopsy, then prolonged digital rectal pressure should be applied. All patients must urinate before leaving the office to assess the presence of hematuria. If a patient has excessive urethral bleeding or is unable to urinate, then a Foley catheter should be inserted. Other possible complications from the biopsy include acute prostatitis and urinary tract infections. The patient should take antibiotics before the biopsy to prevent these complications; however, efficacy does not reach 100%. If a patient does not take antibiotics before coming to the office as instructed, most physicians will

postpone the biopsy because the possible infections, if developed, could lead to full-blown sepsis.

Summary

Prostate cancer is the most prevalent newly diagnosed noncutaneous malignancy in men. With the continued use of PSA screening, there has been a dramatic rise in the number of prostate biopsies performed. TRUS is an essential tool used to detect prostate pathology and perform prostate biopsies.

Box 2: **Protocol for prostate biopsy**

- The patient is placed in a left lateral decubitus position with knees flexed.
- Local anesthesia is administered.
- The probe is set for sagittal and longitudinal views in a dual-screen image.
- A 7-MHz transducer is used, and brightness is set to provide a medium-gray image of the normal peripheral zone.
- Prostate size is measured including height, width, and depth.
- A 12-core systematic biopsy is performed that follows the traditional sextant biopsy, with lateral cores at the base, midgland, and apex from each side. Because the medial cores typically contain transitional zone tissue, the authors do not take additional individual midline samples.

References

[1] Watanabe H, Igari D, Tanahashi Y, et al. Measurements of size and weight of prostate by means of transrectal ultrasonotomography. Tohoku J Exp Med 1974;114:277–85.

[2] Watanabe H, Igari D, Tanahashi Y, et al. Transrectal ultrasonotomography of the prostate. J Urol 1975;114:734–9.

[3] Watanabe H, Igari D, Tanahashi Y, et al. An evaluation of the function of new special equipment for transrectal ultrasonotomography. Tohoku J Exp Med 1976;118:387–92.

[4] Kirby R, McConnell JD, Fitzpatrick JM, et al. Textbook of benign prostatic hyperplasia. Oxford, UK: Oxford University Press; 1996.

[5] Walsh P. Campbell's urology. 8th edition. Philadelphia: Saunders; 2002.

[6] McNeal JE, Redwine EA, Freiha FS, et al. Zonal distribution of prostatic adenocarcinoma.

Correlation with histologic pattern and direction of spread. Am J Surg Pathol 1988;12(12): 897–906.

[7] Wei JT, Calhoun E, Jacobsen SJ. Urologic diseases in America project: benign prostatic hyperplasia. J Urol 2005;173:1256–61.

[8] McNeal JE. The prostate gland: morphology and pathobiology. Monogr Urol 1983;4:3–33.

[9] Lepor H, Nieder A, Feser J, et al. Total prostate and transition zone volumes, and transition zone index are poorly correlated with objective measures of clinical BPH. J Urol 1997;158:85–8.

[10] de la Rosette JJ, van der Schoot DK, Debruyne FM. Recent developments in guidelines on benign prostatic hyperplasia. Curr Opin Urol 2002;12: 3–6.

[11] AUA Practice Guidelines Committee. AUA guideline on management of BPH (2003). Diagnosis and treatment recommendations. J Urol 2003; 170:530–47.

[12] Beckman TJ, Mynderse LA. Evaluation and medical management of benign prostatic hyperplasia. Mayo Clin Proc 2005;80:1356–62.

[13] McConnell JD, Roehrborn CG, Bautista OM, et al, of the Medical Therapy of Prostatic Symptoms (MTOPS) Research Group: the long term effect of doxazosin, finasteride, and combination therapy on the clinical progression of BPH. N Engl J Med 2003;349:2387–98.

[14] Tam PC. Transurethral resection of the prostate: reaffirming the gold standard. Hong Kong Med J 2005;11:79–84.

[15] Gordon NS, Hadlow G, Knight E, et al. Transurethral resection of the prostate: still the gold standard. Aust N Z J Surg 1997;67:354–7.

[16] Jemal A, Murray T, Ward E, et al. Cancer statistics, 2005. CA Cancer J Clin 2005;55:10–30.

[17] Cooperberg MR, Moul JW, Carroll PR. The changing face of prostate cancer. J Clin Oncol 2005;23:8146–51.

[18] Paquette EL, Sun L, Paquette LR, et al. Improved prostate cancer-specific survival and other disease parameters: impact of prostate-specific antigen testing. Urology 2002;60:756–9.

[19] Bauer JJ, Zeng J, Zhang W, et al. Lateral biopsies added to the traditional sextant prostate biopsy pattern increases the detection rate of prostate cancer. Prostate Cancer Prostatic Dis 2000;3: 43–6.

[20] Terris MK. Prostate biopsy strategies: past, present, and future. Urol Clin North Am 2002;29: 205–12.

[21] Richie JP, Catalona WJ, Ahmann FR, et al. Effect of patient age on early detection of prostate cancer with serum prostate-specific antigen and digital rectal examination. Urol 1993;42:365–74.

[22] Wang MC, Valenzuela LA, Murphy GP, et al. Purification of a human prostate specific antigen. Invest Urol 1979;17(2):159–63.

[23] Lilja H. A kallikrein-like serine protease in prostatic fluid cleaves the predominant seminal vesicle protein. J Clin Invest 1985;76(5):1899–903.

[24] Christensson A, Laurell CB, Lilja H. Enzymatic activity of prostate-specific antigen and its reactions with extracellular serine protease inhibitors. Eur J Biochem 1990;194(3):755–63.

[25] Thompson IM, Pauler DK, Goodman PJ, et al. Prevalence of prostate cancer among men with a prostate-specific antigen level < or = 4.0 ng/ml. N Engl J Med 2004;350:2239–46.

[26] Carter HB, Pearson JD, Metter JE, et al. Longitudinal evaluation of prostate specific antigen levels in men with and without prostate disease. JAMA 1992;267:2215–20.

[27] Seaman E, Whang M, Olsson CA, et al. Prostate-specific antigen density: role in patient evaluation and management. Urol Clin North Am 1993;20:653–63.

[28] Christensson A, Bjork T, Nilsson O, et al. Serum PSA complexed to alpha 1-antichymotrypsin as an indicator of prostate cancer. J Urol 1993; 150:100–5.

[29] Catalona WJ, Partin AW, Slawin KM, et al. Use of the percentage of free prostate-specific antigen to enhance differentiation of prostate cancer from benign prostatic disease: a prospective multicenter clinical trial. JAMA 1998;279:1542–7.

[30] Catalona WJ, Bartsch G, Rittenhouse HG, et al. Serum pro-PSA preferentially detects aggressive prostate cancers in men with 2 to 4 ng/ml PSA. J Urol 2004;171:2239–44.

[31] Herget E, Saliken J, Donnelly B, et al. Transrectal ultrasound guided biopsy of the prostate: relation between ASA use and bleeding complications. Can Assoc Radiol J 1999;50:173–6.

[32] Bonow RO, Carabello B, de Leon AC, et al. ACC/ AHA guidelines for the management of patients with valvular heart disease. J Heart Valve Dis 1998;7:672–707.

[33] Davis M, Sofer M, Kim SS, et al. The procedure of transrectal ultrasound guided biopsy of the prostate: a survey of patient preparation and biopsy technique. J Urol 2002;167:566–70.

[34] Carey JM, Korman JH. Transrectal ultrasound guided biopsy of the prostate. Do enemas decrease clinically significant complications? J Urol 2001;166:82–5.

[35] Vallancien G, Prapotnich D, Veillon B, et al. Systematic prostatic biopsies in 100 men with no suspicion of cancer on digital rectal examination. J Urol 1991;146:1308–12.

[36] Gordon PH. Anorectal anatomy and physiology. Gastroenterol Clin North Am 2001;30:1–13.

[37] Shinohara K, Wheeler TM, Scardino PT. The appearance of prostate cancer on transrectal ultrasonography: correlation of imaging and pathological examinations. J Urol 1989;142(1): 76–82.

[38] Brawer MK, Deering RE, Brown M, et al. Predictor of pathologic stage in prostatic carcinoma: the role of neovascularity. Cancer 1994;73: 678–87.

[39] Newman JS, Bree RL, Rubin JM. Prostate cancer: diagnosis with color Doppler sonography with

histologic correlation of each biopsy site. Radiology 1995;195:86–90.

[40] Patel U, Rickards D. The diagnostic value of color Doppler flow in the peripheral zone of the prostate, with histologic correlation. Br J Urol 1994;74:590–5.

[41] Arger PH, Malkowicz B, VanArsdalen KN, et al. Color and power Doppler sonography in the diagnosis of prostate cancer. J Ultrasound Med 2004; 23:623–30.

[42] Pelzer A, Bektic J, Berger AP, et al. Prostate cancer detection in men with PSA 4 to 10 ng/ml using a combined approach of contrast enhanced color Doppler targeted and systematic biopsy. J Urol 2005;173:1926–9.

[43] Ragde H, Kenny GM, Murphy GP, et al. Transrectal ultrasound microbubble contrast angiography of the prostate. Prostate 1997;32:279–83.

[44] Karaman CZ, Unsal A, Akdilli A, et al. The value of contrast enhanced power Doppler ultrasonography in differentiating hypoechoic lesions in the peripheral zone of prostate. Eur J Radiol 2005;54:148–55.

[45] Nash P, Bruce J, Indudhara R, et al. Transrectal ultrasound guided prostatic nerve blockade eases systemic needle biopsy of the prostate. J Urol 1996;155:607–9.

[46] Hodge KK, McNeal JE, Terris MK, et al. Random systematic versus directed ultrasound guided transrectal core biopsies of the prostate. J Urol 1989;142(1):71–4.

[47] Keetch DW, Catalona WJ, Smith DS. Serial prostatic biopsies in men with persistently elevated serum PSA values. J Urol 1994;151(6): 1571–4.

[48] Bauer JJ, Zeng J, Weir J, et al. 3D computer simulated prostate models: lateral prostate biopsies increase the detection rate of prostate cancer. Urology 1999;53(5):961–7.

[49] Chen ME, Troncoso P, Johnston DA, et al. Optimization of prostate biopsy strategy using computer based analysis. J Urol 1997;158(6): 2168–75.

[50] Ravery V, Goldblatt L, Royer B, et al. Extensive biopsy protocol improves the detection rate of prostate cancer. J Urol 2000;164(2):393–6.

[51] Norberg M, Egevad L, Holmberg L, et al. The sextant protocol for ultrasound-guided core biopsies of the prostate underestimates the presence of cancer. Urology 1997;50(4): 562–6.

[52] Epstein JI, Walsh PC, Carter HB. Importance of posterolateral needle biopsies in the detection of prostate cancer. Urology 2001;57:1112–6.

[53] Naughton CK, Miller DC, Mager DE, et al. A prospective randomized trial comparing 6 versus 12 prostate biopsy cores: impact on cancer detection. J Urol 2000;164:388.

[54] Jones JS, Oder M, Zippe CD. Saturation prostate biopsy with periprostatic block can be performed in the office. J Urol 2002;168(5): 2108–19.

RADIOLOGIC
CLINICS
OF NORTH AMERICA

Radiol Clin N Am 44 (2006) 689–710

Benign Prostatic Hyperplasia: A Review and Ultrasound Classification

Neil F. Wasserman, MD

- Initial clinical assessment of benign prostatic hyperplasia
- Initial assessment with imaging
- Urologic management
- Anatomy of the prostate
- Pathogenesis and clinical effects of benign prostatic hyperplasia
- Appearance of benign prostatic hyperplasia on transrectal ultrasound
- Methods of estimating prostate size
- Prostatic contour
- Ultrasound classification of benign prostatic hyperplasia
- Postoperative changes
- Acknowledgments
- References

In the United States, the prevalence of lower urinary tract symptoms (LUTS) is 31% to 36% in men aged 60 to 69 years and 44% in men 70 years and older [1]. Mean life expectancy worldwide is 64 years; the number of men over age 65 years (currently 380 million) is projected to increase to 680 million by 2020 [2]. The Director General of the World Health Organization reminds us "increased longevity without quality of life is an empty promise. Health expectancy is at least as important as life expectancy" [2]. Histopathologic benign prostatic hyperplasia (BPH) is age dependent. Early development usually occurs after age 40 years [3]; by age 60 years, its prevalence is greater than 50% and by age 85 years, it is as much as 90%. About 50% of men who have a histologic diagnosis of BPH have moderate to severe LUTS [4]. Traditionally, any symptoms produced by a variety of abnormal

conditions of the prostate have been referred to as "prostatism." New and more precise terminology in current use is listed in Box 1 [5]. Another term used in this discussion of BPH is *the standard patient*, which refers to a man (usually older than 50 years) who (1) has LUTS, (2) is consulting a qualified health care provider, and (3) does not have known prostate cancer, diabetes, diabetic neuropathy, a history suggesting neurologic disorder, history of pelvic surgery or trauma, or previously unsuccessful treatment for LUTS [6].

The purpose of this article is to briefly review the current general clinical management of patients presenting to their primary care physician or urologist with symptoms of LUTS and the role of medical imaging in the pretreatment assessment and management of these men. Emphasis is placed on the assessment of BPH on transrectal ultrasound

I have no relationship with any commercial company that has a direct financial interest in the subject matter or materials discussed in this article or with a company making a competing product. I am not a consultant for any related companies, nor do I own stock or have any equity interests or patent-licensing agreements.
Department of Radiology 114, Department of Veterans Affairs Medical Center, 1 Veterans Drive, Minneapolis, MN 55417, USA
E-mail address: wasse001@umn.edu

doi:10.1016/j.rcl.2006.07.005

(TRUS) of the prostate and the use of this modality for pretreatment evaluation for open and transurethral resection of the prostate (TURP) or minimally invasive therapy. The appearance of BPH on CT and MR imaging is mentioned. MR imaging and MR spectrographic findings are not discussed.

Initial clinical assessment of benign prostatic hyperplasia

When the patient initially presents to the clinician, the first determination is whether to treat the patient's symptoms. This decision cannot be made until a thorough medical history, physical examination, symptom scoring, uroflow, and limited laboratory tests are performed [7].

Medical history must identify the presence of other potential etiologies of voiding dysfunction, such as urinary tract infection including prostatitis, neurologic disorders such as diabetes mellitus, Parkinson's disease, and multiple sclerosis causing neurogenic bladder, and prostate carcinoma.

The physical examination should include a careful neurologic assessment and digital rectal examination to rule out nodules suspicious for cancer and to estimate prostate size. Estimation of prostate size on digital rectal examination or clinical endoscopy is accurate only for volumes up to 40 cm^3 [8].

Symptom scoring through self-administered questionnaires has arguably become the most important determinate for decision making regarding whether to treat LUTS. Two scoring scales (the American Urological Association Symptom Index and the International Prostate Symptom Score) are validated for a variety of ethnic, racial, and language-speaking populations. The maximum sum score for symptoms using seven questions on each scale is 35. Most clinicians also have the patient fill out a global estimate of urinary quality of life using a questionnaire that rates quality from 0 (best) to 5 (worst). These tools are useful supplements to the unstructured interview to establish baseline patient discomfort and to follow the patient's symptoms over time.

Uroflow study requires the patient to void into the toilet through a funnel equipped with a flow meter. The patient is asked to activate the flowmeter at the onset of voiding and to turn it off at the end of voiding. A strip chart is produced with graphic documentation of peak velocity of urine flow in milliliters per second, the slope of the rise in velocity, and the length of the voiding cycle (Fig. 1). Normal peak velocity is above 15 mL/s, whereas severe obstruction or detrusor insufficiency is likely present when peak velocity is 10 mL/s or less. Bladder outlet obstruction (BOO) is characterized by a shallow initial slope to a low peak velocity and by delayed return to baseline at the end of the voiding cycle (see Fig. 1B). It is unfortunate that these results are not specific for BPH and are mimicked by primary bladder dysfunction due to neurologic disorders and other conditions (such as prostatitis) producing infravesical obstruction, even in the absence of such findings in the medical history and physical examination. An abnormal uroflow (flow rate) study is usually taken to indicate BOO likely due to BPH. When medical conditions obscure interpretation of the uroflow examination, the more definitive but invasive urodynamic (pressure-flow) studies may be indicated to make actual measurements of infravesical pressure during voiding and to delineate abnormal patterns of detrusor contraction. Because urodynamic tests are labor intensive, expensive, and invasive, they are not commonly done during early investigation of LUTS.

Initial laboratory tests include urinalysis for blood and infection and serum prostate-specific antigen to screen for prostate cancer. Urine cytology is reserved for men who are at risk for bladder carcinoma in situ that can cause irritative bladder symptoms. Serum creatinine is not initially recommended in the standard patient who has LUTS.

An endoscopic procedure (urethrocystoscopy) is not considered part of the initial assessment in the standard patient. It is an option when the decision for surgery has been made or when initial assessment discovers evidence suggesting tumor, renal failure, urolithiasis, or a history of previous urologic surgical procedures.

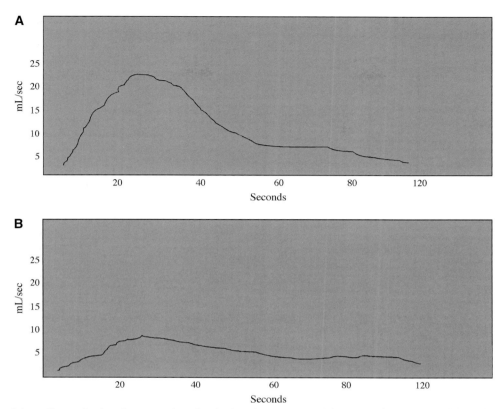

Fig. 1. (*A*) Uroflow strip showing normal peak velocity of 22.5 mL/s and duration of micturition. (*B*) Uroflow strip showing low peak velocity and delayed voiding due to infravesical obstruction.

Initial assessment with imaging

No initial imaging is recommended in the standard patient [6,7]. If the initial clinical assessment discovers that the patient has a complicating disorder potentially affecting the upper urinary tract, then intravenous urography, renal ultrasound, or CT may be needed, whether or not intervention is required for LUTS (Table 1). When a decision is made to treat the patient with surgery or a minimally invasive procedure, imaging becomes an important option and constitutes the balance of this article's discussion.

Urologic management

The initial assessment assigns the patient to one of two categories: mild symptoms with minimally obstructive uroflow or moderate to severe symptoms with obstructive uroflow. Patients who have a symptom score of 7 or less and patients who have a moderate or severe symptom score of 8 or greater whose symptoms are not bothersome and do not interfere with their everyday life should be managed by watchful waiting, limiting of fluid intake at bedtime, and decreasing caffeine and alcohol intake.

For those who have moderate to severe symptoms and have not developed complications of BPH such as renal insufficiency, urinary retention, or recurrent infection, options include watchful waiting, medical therapies, and minimally invasive or surgical therapies [7].

Medical and minimally invasive therapeutic techniques are recommended for men who have moderate to severe symptoms with abnormal uroflow whose quality of life is significantly affected and who desire treatment. The most commonly selected treatment is medical management with α-adrenergic blocking agents or 5α-reductase inhibitors.

Other optional therapies include thermal therapies, transurethral needle ablation that uses radiofrequency energy, laser, and high-intensity focused ultrasound to shrink the enlarged lateral lobes (transition zone [TZ]) of the prostate. The details of these treatments are beyond the scope of this review. How the selection of one of these options may invoke the use of ultrasound imaging is discussed later in this article.

Currently, open surgery, TURP, transurethral electrovaporization (TUEVP), and transurethral incision of the prostate are reserved for men who have moderately severe to severe symptoms with

Table 1: **Initial assessment or secondary findings indicating imaging studies**

Finding	Imaging study
Hematuria	IVU or CT urogram
Abnormal DRE	TRUS with biopsy
Elevated PSA	TRUS with biopsy
Elevated serum creatinine	Renal US, CT abdomen/ pelvis
Urinary retention	Renal US or US for prostate volume

Abbreviations: DRE, digital rectal examination; IVU, intravenous urography; PSA, prostate-specific antingen; US, ultrasound.
From Koyanagi T, Artibani W, Correa R, et al. Initial diagnostic evaluation of men with lower urinary tract symptoms. In: Denis L, Griffiths K, Khoury S, et al, editors. 4th International Consultation on Benign Prostatic Hyperplasia, Paris, July 2–5, 1997. Plymoth, UK: Plymbridge Distributors Ltd; 1998. p. 183–4.

signs of obstruction and for those showing the complications of obstruction mentioned earlier. A preoperative assessment with imaging may be requested by the urologic surgeon.

Anatomy of the prostate

To understand how the anatomic changes of BPH influence voiding function, we must consider that the prostate is not only a glandular organ but also a very muscular organ. Abnormal effects on the anatomy may influence either or both of these anatomic systems, and the interaction of glandular and stromal hyperplasia may determine the success of management strategies.

The glandular anatomy has been thoroughly discussed by McNeal [9–12]. The prostate is divided into four glandular zones (peripheral, central, transition, periurethral) and one stromal zone (anterior fibromuscular stroma) (Fig. 2). A small zone of periurethral glandular tissue is found primarily

behind the proximal prostatic urethra (also known as preprostatic urethra). These periurethral glands (PUG) are divided into two important groups that influence the lobar pattern of prostate enlargement when undergoing BPH. There is a superficial group of PUG in the immediate submucosa of the proximal prostatic urethra directly opening into the lumen and a deep group of PUG between the mucosa and inner longitudinal muscle layer emptying through long ducts into the urethra just above the verumontanum (Fig. 3). This distinction is discussed later in this article. An understanding of the zonal anatomy of the prostate is fundamental to an appreciation of the gross and imaging changes seen in everyday practice.

The descriptions of the stromal anatomy of the prostate described in the following summary are discussed in detail in other studies and reviews [13–17]. The stromal anatomy (Fig. 4A) includes fibromuscular extensions of the detrusor muscle of the bladder, enveloping the upper prostate anteriorly, posteriorly, and laterally. The striated muscle of the membranous urethra (external sphincter) and pelvic floor extend upward to encase the inferior one third of the outer prostate, interdigitating with the extentions of the detrusor muscle above to form the outer aspect of the prostatic capsule and the anterior fibromuscular stroma described by McNeal [9–12]. These tissues combine with compressed lamellar fibrostroma from within the prostate and together compose the outer "capsule" of the prostate. Some anatomists object to the term *capsule* because it is not easily stripped away from the parenchyma, but the term is in general use [18].

The proximal prostatic urethra is composed of mucosa, submucosa, and two smooth muscle layers derived from inferior extension of the deep muscle of the trigone. These muscles end near the verumontanum, a mound of smooth muscle on the posterior wall of the prostatic urethra through which the ejaculatory ducts empty into the urethra.

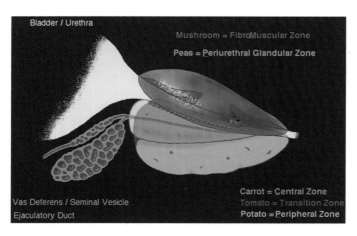

Fig. 2. Illustration showing the normal zonal anatomy of the prostate depicted with mnemonics based on the first letters of vegetables.

Bladder / Urethra

Mushroom = FibroMuscular Zone

Peas = Periurethral Glandular Zone

Carrot = Central Zone
Tomato = Transition Zone
Potato = Peripheral Zone

Vas Deferens / Seminal Vesicle
Ejaculatory Duct

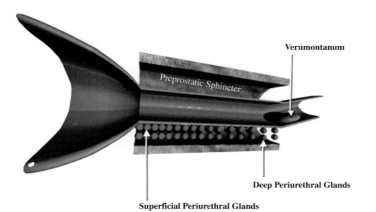

Verumontanum

Preprostatic Sphincter

Deep Periurethral Glands

Superficial Periurethral Glands

Fig. 3. Illustration showing retroure-thral superficial and deep PUG between the submucosa and the inner longitudinal muscular layer of the preprostatic (proximal prostatic) urethra. Note the greater abundance of PUG proximally near the bladder neck.

The outer circular smooth muscle of the proximal urethra is open anteriorly, fanning downward and anteriorly to blend with the muscle of the anterior fibromuscular stroma (see Fig. 4). The continuous muscles of the bladder neck and proximal urethra are together variously termed the *internal sphincter* or the *vesicourethral sphincter*.

There is striated muscle surrounding the lower third of the prostatic urethra (also known as the postprostatic urethra) below the verumontanum. This represents an upward extension of the pelvic muscles of the urogenital diaphragm. The membranous urethra is surrounded from the outside by (1) the slow-twitch striated muscles of the so-called "urogenital diaphragm" (voluntary muscles of the pelvic floor), sometimes termed the *extrinsic sphincter*; (2) an outer longitudinal muscle sphincter with a mixture of striated and smooth muscle that is a complex mixture of slow- and fast-twitch fibers;

and (3) an inner circular fast-twitch smooth muscle. These latter two layers of muscle are referred to as the *intrinsic sphincter*. Together, this area is considered the external urethral sphincter and the primary zone responsible for continence in men. When there is voluntary contraction of the external sphincter under TRUS observation, one can visualize the overall sphincteric effect on the prostatic apex as it is elevated and squeezed.

Bridging the space between the fibromuscular outer capsule and the inner core of urethral muscle is a latticework of fibromuscular stroma supporting the glandular and ductal elements of the prostate (see Fig. 4). When one examines how all of these stromal muscular structures interconnect from the bladder to the pelvic floor, one can understand how an increased muscle tone can result in BOO and urethral obstruction, even without significant hyperplasia of the glandular regions (Fig. 5).

Pathogenesis and clinical effects of benign prostatic hyperplasia

A full discussion of the complex interactions between extrinsic and intrinsic factors leading to

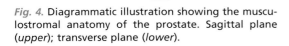

Symphisis

Bladder

Preprostatic sphinc.
Prostatic sphinc.
Ext. sphinc.

Fibromuscular layer

Capsule

Urethral sphincter

Fig. 4. Diagrammatic illustration showing the musculostromal anatomy of the prostate. Sagittal plane (*upper*); transverse plane (*lower*).

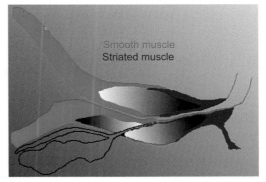

Smooth muscle
Striated muscle

Fig. 5. Stylized sagittal illustration showing smooth and striated muscle distribution from bladder base to the urogenital diaphragm.

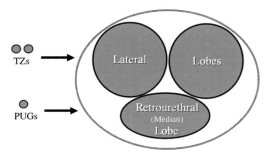

Fig. 6. Illustration showing the relationship between zones and lobes. With the development of BPH, the TZ becomes distinct lobes bounded by stroma and the PUG evolve into the retrourethral (median) lobe.

prostatic glandular and stromal hyperplasia is too large a topic to be reviewed here but is nicely summarized elsewhere [19]. There is direct evidence of an inflammatory role in patients developing symptoms from BPH [20].

A large body of knowledge has demonstrated that there are two major tissues that undergo hyperplasia in the prostate [21–27]. All investigations emphasize that hyperplasia occurs in glandular (epithelial) and stromal tissues, the latter including muscular fibers. There is some controversy regarding what the stromal/epithelial ratio is in symptomatic patients, but most investigations suggest that stromal hyperplasia dominates. Massive disproportionate epithelial hyperplasia results in marked enlargement in the glandular tissues of the prostate, increasing the bulk and producing potential obstruction by compressive mechanical narrowing of the bladder neck and urethra (referred to as the *static* effect). Obstruction caused by hyperplasia or

increased tone of the musculostroma is termed the *dynamic* mechanism of obstruction by BPH. Frequently, a component of both mechanisms operates to produce obstructive symptoms and signs. It has been shown that random biopsies of the prostate such as would be obtained by TRUS guidance are representative of the stromal/epithelial ratio throughout the prostate [26,27].

Although the earliest microscopic signs of BPH begin in the PUG posterior to the proximal urethra in the fourth decade [11], micronodular growth soon begins to predominate in the TZ. Progressive TZ hyperplasia produces a growth in the number of nodules anterolateral to the urethra. These tiny nodules grow in size and coalesce into ever-larger nodules. Because the glands of the TZ are distributed between the urethral smooth muscle fibers, they become encased in stroma and, with macroscopic growth, stretch these muscle bundles around the nests of hyperplastic glands. As the coalescent glandular tissue expands, the surrounding stroma becomes compressed, producing a distinct demarcation at which stage the bilateral hyperplastic TZ tissues can be accurately called the "lateral lobes."

If there is continued growth of the PUG, the resulting well-demarcated expanding midline retrourethral tissue is referred to as the "median lobe" (Fig. 6). This growth occurs in a potential retrourethral inverted pyramidal space between the urethra

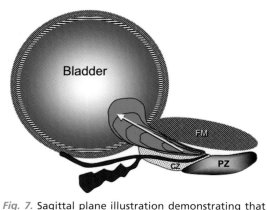

Fig. 7. Sagittal plane illustration demonstrating that retrourethral (median lobe) hyperplasia (*pea green*) is greater in volume proximally. Because the potential space between the urethra and CZ is an inverted pyramid, the vector of growth favors a path of least resistance in the proximal direction (*arrow*). FM, fibromuscular zone; PZ, peripheral zone.

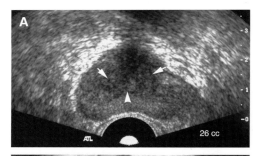

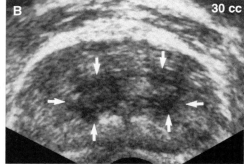

Fig. 8. Earliest changes of TZ BPH. (*A*) Axial TRUS image showing coarse hypoechoic areas (*arrows*) immediately anterolateral to the verumontanum (*arrowhead*), representing first visible sign of TZ BPH. (*B*) Progressive early TZ BPH (*arrows*).

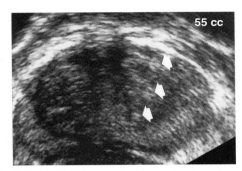

Fig. 9. Axial TRUS image showing 3- to 5-mm hyperechoic grossly visible nodules (*arrowheads*), likely stromal.

and the central zone (CZ), with its apex immediately above the level of the verumontanum and its base behind the bladder neck. As growth of the periurethral glandular zone continues, it meets resistance below by the convergence of surrounding tissues at the verumontanum resulting in a growth vector in the upward direction along a course of least resistance toward the area behind the bladder neck (Fig. 7). All of the macroscopic changes described previously can be described by a carefully performed and interpreted TRUS examination of the prostate.

A little-appreciated fact is that although BPH predominates in the inner gland (TZ and periurethral glandular zone), it also involves the peripheral zone (PZ) [28–31]. BPH may account for up to 58% of individuals who have had biopsies performed for a hypoechoic PZ nodule [32].

Appearance of benign prostatic hyperplasia on transrectal ultrasound

The earliest visible ultrasound finding of BPH can be seen in the fourth decade as symmetric, predominantly homogeneous hypoechoic spherical areas just superior and anterolateral to the verumontanum (Fig. 8). With growth, these tissues of the anterior paraurethral TZ region become more variable in appearance but remain hypoechoic. Homogeneity progresses to a mixed heterogeneous pattern. Additional TZ growth results in diffusely heterogeneous or multinodular 2- to 5-mm isoechoic foci superimposed on a hypoechoic background (Fig. 9). These foci represent the coalescence of smaller foci into more distinct larger ones. Continued enlargement produces fusion of these isoechoic nodules into macronodules 1 to 2 cm in size (Fig. 10). Hasegawa and colleagues [33] studied the internal echo patterns of BPH and compared their appearance with open prostatectomy tissues. They reported two distinct patterns. A fine echogenic pattern was histologically associated with small cystic atrophic

glands less than 1.5 mm in diameter, and a "rough" echopenic pattern was caused by larger cystic atrophic glands 1.5 mm or greater. Blockage of prostatic ducts by stromal hyperplasia may produce cystic dilation of the glands of the TZ that can be extensive in larger adenomas (usually measuring 2 to 10 mm in diameter) and easily resolved by ultrasound (Fig. 11).

A hypoechoic band of compressed fibromuscular stroma, often referred to as the "surgical capsule," represents the advancing perimeter of the adenoma. This structure is the compressed outer smooth muscle of the urethra (see Fig. 12). Total volume of TZ growth may be symmetric or asymmetric, producing enough outward impression on the PZ to compress it into a thin rind of tissue outside the surgical capsule and to distort the prostatic contour. Asymmetric hyperplasia may be palpated as asymmetric enlargement, leading to a request for ultrasound (see Fig. 12).

TRUS is not recommended in the initial evaluation of LUTS; however, the American Urological Association recommends ultrasound as an optional test in patients in whom invasive therapies are contemplated [7]. Ultrasound measurements can predict the natural history and progression of LUTS and BPH and the therapeutic response to medical

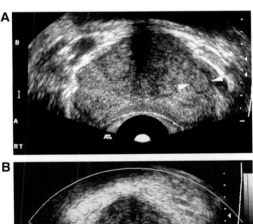

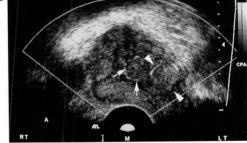

Fig. 10. (A) Axial TRUS image showing 5-mm isoechoic grossly visible nodules outlined by compressed hypoechoic stroma (*arrowheads*). (B) Axial color flow Doppler TRUS image showing coalescence of smaller nodules into larger 1- to 2-cm ones (*arrows, arrowheads*). Note the vascular structures displaced about the left nodule.

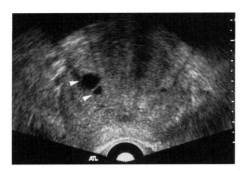

Fig. 11. Axial TRUS image demonstrating two typical benign cysts in the hyperplastic TZ (*arrowheads*).

management. The ratio of TZ to total prostate volume (TZ index) has been shown to correlate with symptom scores for LUTS and with urodynamic measures of urine flow and detrusor pressure [34,35] and can predict response to medical management with 5α-reductase inhibitors [36]. The minimal description in the radiologist's TRUS report must include the size, contour, and lobar distribution of prostatic growth.

Methods of estimating prostate size

There is a large body of evidence attesting to the accuracy of transrectal, transabdominal, and transperineal ultrasound for prostate volume calculation [37–39]. Because the specific gravity of prostate tissue is nearly the same as for water, volume is roughly equivalent to prostatic weight. A variety of methods have been used to measure volume, including serial planimetry, three-dimensional imaging, and simple calculations from orthogonal ultrasound-based measurements using geometric models such as the formula for a sphere or prolate ellipsoid.

The serial planimetric volume method is the most labor intensive of techniques to measure prostate volume in vivo. It involves special step-section instrumentation wherein the ultrasound probe is inserted to a point above the base and retracted by exact, 5-mm increments through the transverse planes of the gland to a level through the apex. At each stop, a circumference line is drawn electronically and an area is calculated by the software. After all sections are measured, the software calculates

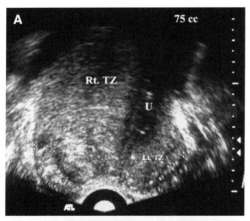

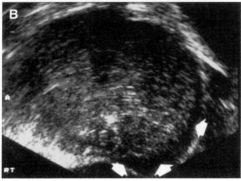

Fig. 12. Axial TRUS images showing that BPH growth of the TZ can be asymmetric. (*A*) Right-sided (Rt.) TZ hyperplasia displaces urethra (U) toward the left (Lt.). (*B*) Asymmetric left TZ hyperplasia produces a pronounced palpable prominence on digital rectal examination (*arrowheads*), which is often mistaken for malignant tumor on physical examination.

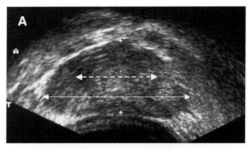

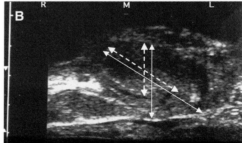

Fig. 13. TRUS-guided measurement of the prostate based on the prolate ellipsoid model. (*A*) Axial view showing the total transverse measurement (*solid line*) and measurement of the adenomatous growth (*dashed line*). (*B*) Longitudinal view showing total measurement (*solid lines*) and adenomatous measurements (*dashed lines*) for length and anteroposterior diameter.

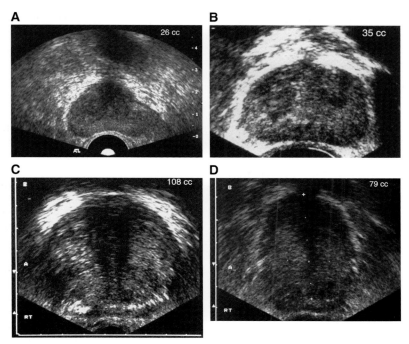

Fig. 14. Axial TRUS images showing changes in prostate contour with growth. (*A*) Nearly normal triangular contour demonstrating predominant PZ tissue with only minimal hypoechoic early TZ hyperplasia. (*B*) Mild TZ hyperplasia showing transverse oval shape as the paired TZ hyperplasia begins to fill out the anterolateral contour. (*C*) Further TZ enlargement produces a nearly round axial contour. (*D*) High intracapsular pressure with "trapped" growing adenoma causes disproportionate AP oval shape because the anterior fibromuscular stroma has less elastic recoil than the posterior and lateral prostatic capsule.

the volume of each 5-mm slab and summates the volumes to achieve the total prostatic volume.

Three-dimensional methods have been shown experimentally to be accurate but are even more technique dependent and labor intensive and, thus, rarely performed in the field. The same is true of CT and MR techniques.

The prolate ellipsoid model is the de facto standard for the calculation of prostate volume and uses the following formula: transverse diameter × anteroposterior diameter × length × 0.52. These dimensions are measured by caliper during TRUS. The software programmed on most machines calculates the volume (Fig. 13). The anteroposterior diameter (AP) is most accurately measured with end-fire probes in the sagittal plane to avoid the "salami" distortion of measurements in the axial plane. Measurement is made for the total volume of the prostate and the inner tissues, usually hyperplastic TZ.

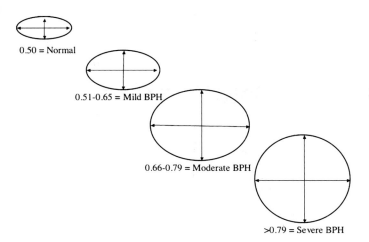

0.50 = Normal

0.51–0.65 = Mild BPH

0.66–0.79 = Moderate BPH

>0.79 = Severe BPH

Fig. 15. Diagrammatic illustrations of the use of the AP-to-transverse ratio as viewed in the axial TRUS plane to suggest a numeric value describing the shape of the prostate. Patients with a ratio of 0.80 or greater show good correlation with uroflow and symptom scores indicating obstruction. These patients also have a better probability of responding to treatment.

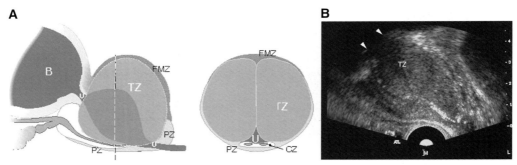

Fig. 16. Trapping of TZ. Diagrammatic illustration (*A*) and sagittal TRUS image (*B*) showing "trapping" of the enlarging TZ with increased intraprostatic pressure causing disproportional increase of AP diameter. The bladder neck (*arrowheads*) is competent, preventing decompressive herniation of the adenoma into the bladder. B, bladder; CZ, central zone; FMZ, fibromuscular zone; PZ, peripheral zone; TZ, transition zone; U, urethra.

Why does size count? After the decision is made for therapeutic intervention, accurate BPH volume measurement is important for several reasons. When invasive surgery is considered, the urologist is limited to open resection if the prostate volume exceeds his personal threshold of comfort based on technical skill and speed. Most surgeons consider prostatic volume greater than 75 cm^3 an indication for open resection and favor TURP when the volume is less than 75 cm^3 [40]. The most experienced and skillful resectionists may extend TURP to over 100 cm^3, but prolonged resection times are associated with complications of bleeding, fluid intoxication, and urethral and bladder neck strictures. If the prostate is less than 30 cm^3 in volume, especially in a younger man, transurethral incision of the prostate (TUIP) at the level of the bladder neck is quicker and an effective treatment, resulting is less risk of retrograde ejaculation [41,42]. Manufacturer-recommended size limits exist for all microwave thermotherapy devices [7], and an upper limit of 60 cm^3 is recommended for treatment

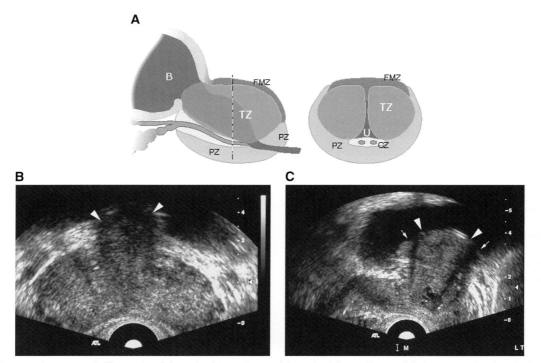

Fig. 17. Diagrammatic illustration (*A*), sagittal TRUS image (*B*), and axial TRUS image (*C*) demonstrating herniation of the TZ (*arrowheads*) through an incompetent bladder neck (*arrows*) partially decompressing high intraprostatic pressure. B, bladder; CZ, central zone; FMZ, fibromuscular zone; PZ, peripheral zone; TZ, transition zone; U, urethra.

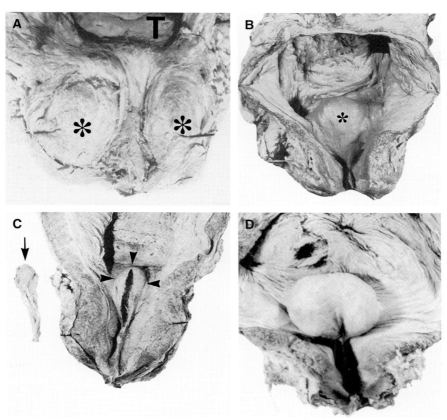

Fig. 18. (A) Photograph of gross prostate specimen from the front following anterior midline incision through the anterior urethral wall and pinning back of the opened tissues. Bilateral TZ hyperplasia (*asterisks*) is demonstrated. T, trigone. (B) Photograph of specimen showing Randall's commissural hyperplasia (*asterisk*). (C) Photograph of small Albarrán's lobe (*arrow*) shelled out from overlying thin layer of uroepithelial mucosa (*arrowheads*) demonstrating the long pedicle detached from the posterior wall of the preprostatic urethra above the verumontanum. (D) Photograph of a more developed Albarrán's lobe within the bladder neck. (*Adapted from* Randall A. Surgical pathology of prostatic obstructions. Baltimore (MD): Williams & Wilkins; 1931.)

with radiofrequency transurethral needle ablation devices [7]. Side-firing laser prostatectomy may not be indicated in men who have a prostate larger than 30 cm³ in some circumstances [43].

Size considerations also play a role in selection of medical management. Treatment with 5α-reductase inhibitors, which act by shrinking hyperplastic glandular tissue, are less effective in reducing the static effects of obstruction in patients who have prostate volumes less than 50 cm³ [44]. Total length measurement of the urethra encased by adenoma is also of interest to the urologist when selecting sizes of ablative instruments and for placement of stents.

Although knowledge of prostate size is valuable in treatment planning and follow-up of BPH, size alone should not be a factor in the decision to treat BPH or LUTS [6]. When performed before surgery, TRUS provides urologists with an accurate estimate of TZ and median lobe volume, a more pertinent

measurement than total prostate volume when potential blood loss and other complications related to operative time are considered [45].

Prostatic contour

Before grossly apparent hyperplasia, the prostate has a triangular shape and volume less than 15 cm³ and is composed anteriorly of the hypoechoic vesicourethral sphincter and posteriorly of the PZ and, to a lesser extent, the CZ (Fig. 14A) [26,44]. By the fifth decade, early BPH in the anteriorly located TZ begins to bilaterally distend the anterior contour, producing an ellipsoid profile (see Fig. 14B). Because the posterior and lateral prostatic capsule have less elasticity than the anterior fibromuscular stroma, there is more resistance to transverse enlargement, and further growth of the TZ disproportionately increases the AP diameter.

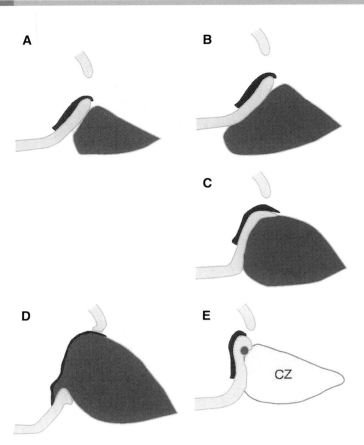

Therefore, as BPH progresses, the ellipsoid shape becomes less oval and more rounded (see Fig. 14C). Ultimately, the AP diameter may exceed the transverse diameter (see Fig.14D). Globularization produced by the disproportionate growth in the AP direction is accompanied by thinning of the anterior fibromuscular stroma; however, the latter cannot be resolved from TZ hyperplasia with ultrasound. These changes were quantitated with ultrasound measurements and described as the presumed circle area ratio (PCAR) [35]. PCAR is measured on TRUS at the transverse level of greatest apparent area. It is calculated as the ratio of the measured area at this level to the area of a presumed circle of which the circumference is equal to the maximum circumference of the prostate on horizontal section. It has been shown that a PCAR ratio greater than 0.80 strongly correlates with urodynamic measurement of infravesical obstruction [35]. Other ultrasound-based indices including TZ volume and the ratio of TZ volume to total prostate volume (TZ index) may predict peak flow and correlate with improvement in peak flow with treatment of BPH with 5α-reductase inhibitors [36]. The ratio of the maximal anteroposterior to maximal transverse diameter (prostatic ratio) also correlates with symptom scoring, and is a simple, easily performed proxy for PCAR [34].

The progression of shapes—from triangular to transverse to transverse ovoid axis to round to AP ovoid axis—clearly correlates to the ratio of these diameters (Fig. 15).

The shape of the enlarging prostate is also influenced by the elastic properties of the capsule and fibromuscular stroma in any given patient and whether the bladder neck remains competent or the enlarging lateral lobes (TZ) herniate through the vesicourethral sphincter. If the hyperplastic lobes are "trapped" below the bladder neck and elastic recoil of the capsule is strong, then intracapsular pressure would be expected to rise rapidly, producing symptoms and signs of obstruction. This increased intracapsular pressure is reflected in the increased AP diameter of the prostate relative to the transverse measurement because the anterior fibromuscular stroma has less elastic recoil properties compared with the capsule and, thus, less resistance to expansion under the influence of TZ growth (Fig. 16). In contrast, if there is relative incompetence of the bladder neck, then upward herniation of the growing TZ results in less pressure on the anterior fibromuscular stroma and less apparent increase in the AP diameter (Fig. 17).

Ultrasound classification of benign prostatic hyperplasia

In 1931, Randall proposed a gross pathologic classification of BPH based on careful observations made in 222 postmortem cases (Box 2) [46]. His classic treatise describes the lobar distributions seen by making an anterior incision in the midline through the en bloc bladder and prostatic specimen. The incision line is pinned back laterally, thereby exposing the sagittal surfaces of the anterior prostate, the open posterior urethra, the trigone, and the interior surface of the urinary bladder (Fig. 18A). The posterior midline components of the prostate were viewed indirectly by their impressions or displacements of the posterior urethral wall and trigone. Randall [46] studiously correlated these patterns with available clinical records on these patients and recorded simple descriptive statistics regarding age and comorbid conditions. There have been no further attempts to classify the gross patterns of prostatic growth. It is unfortunate that his work, although highly regarded at the time, faded into obscurity. A very brief and more recent summary of Randall's work was published in 1983 [47]. The validity of many of Randall's [46] descriptions is untainted by time; however, his observations were largely limited to a description of surface gross anatomy. With the development of high-resolution endorectal ultrasound, clinicians are now able to evaluate the internal anatomy of the prostate. Better yet, this can be done in vivo and the information gained can be used to diagnose and treat prostatic disorders.

Any modern classification must consider advanced knowledge regarding the pathophysiology of bladder neck obstruction and BPH in addition to the diagnosis and treatment of the latter.

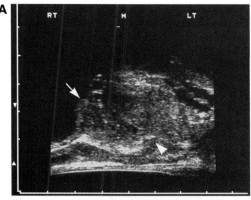

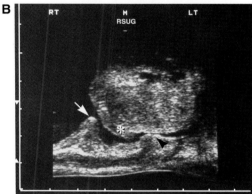

Fig. 20. Prominent posterior vesical lip. (*A*) Sagittal TRUS image demonstrates prominent posterior vesical lip, not to be confused with retrourethral (median lobe) hyperplasia or fibrous median bar. Arrowhead points to entry of the ejaculatory duct into the verumontanum. (*B*) Sagittal saline retrograde urethrogram in the same patient better demonstrating the prominent posterior vesical lip (*arrow*). The verumontanum is also indicated (*black arrowhead*). Note the hyperplastic TZ nodule protruding into the urethra (*asterisk*).

> *Box 2:* **Randall classification of benign prostatic hypertrophy**
>
> Type I Simple bilateral lobe (Fig. 1)
> Type II Solitary posterior commissural (Fig. 2)
> Type III Bilateral and commissural (Fig. 3)
> Type IV Solitary subcervical (Albarrán's) lobe (Fig. 4A)
> Type V Bilateral and subcervical lobe (Fig. 4B)
> Type VI Bilateral, subcervical, and commissural
> Type VII Anterior
> Type VIII Subtrigonal lobe
>
> *Data from* Randall A. Surgical pathology of prostatic obstructions. Baltimore (MD): Williams & Wilkins; 1931.

McNeal's [9] descriptions of microscopic zonal anatomy have largely replaced older concepts of lobar anatomy. With pathologic growth, the TZ becomes well delineated, compressing the outer circular muscle layer of the urethra into a fibrostromal pseudocapsule (the surgical capsule). In this pathologic state, these hyperplastic zones may be aptly referred to as "lobes." The TZ becomes a lateral lobe and the bulky PUG hyperplasia becomes a midline retrourethral or pedunculated intraurethral lobar structure. Occasionally, an area of ectopic PUG enlarges high in the subtrigonal region.

Randall's [46] designation of the tissue posterior to the proximal urethra as "commissural" reflected his opinion that it represented hyperplastic extension of the lateral lobes across the posterior midline (see Fig. 18B). As a result of modern histologic descriptions by McNeal and others, it would be appropriate to generically rename this tissue as "ret-rourethral." Randall adopted Albarrán's term *subcervical* for adenomas arising from the superficial PUG in the posterior wall of the proximal urethra, which with intralumenal growth become pedunculated (see Fig. 18C, D). For simplicity, the term *pedunculated* was chosen for the ultrasound classification of this pattern.

In a careful review of 100 TRUS studies (Neil F. Wasserman, MD, unpublished data, July 2001), it was found that the Randall classification was inadequate to fully describe the spectrum of changes observed and, to be relevant to practical clinical patient management, some modification was required (Box 3 and Table 2). Particular difficulty was encountered in this attempt at ultrasound classification of BPH in describing the variations of posterior midline enlargements (Fig. 19). The first difficulty was in distinguishing enlargements posterior to the proximal urethra from those within and above the urethra (pedunculated). The second issue was how to deal with the presence of bladder neck

Table 2: Comparison of Randall and ultrasound classifications of benign prostatic hyperplasia

Randall	Ultrasound
I Simple bilateral	1 Bilateral TZ
II Solitary commissural	2 Retrourethral
III Bilateral/commissural	3 Bilateral/retrourethral
IV Solitary subcervical	4 Solitary /multiple pedunculated
V Bilateral/subcervical	5 Bilateral/pedunculated
VI Bilateral/subcervical/commissural	6 Subtrigonal
VII Anterior	7 Other combinations

Data from Randall A. Surgical pathology of prostatic obstructions. Baltimore (MD): Williams & Wilkins; 1931.

herniation of this tissue, which because of its propensity to spread the decussating longitudinal muscle fibers of the detrusor, is more likely to produce physiologic effects. Turner-Warwick [16] believed that a muscular ring formed by the bladder neck was induced by underlying detrusor dyssynergia to produce the prominent posterior vesical lip so often noted in that condition (Fig. 20). He pointed out that this condition might be subclinical and occur earlier in life than BPH. He further suggested that subsequent hyperplasia in the upper midline posterior to the urethra below this muscular ring may prevent the adenoma from decompressing through the bladder neck and thereby cause it to become "trapped" within the prostatic capsule. Randall [46], however, believed that the development of focal glandular hyperplasia immediately posterior to the bladder neck stimulated nearby hypertrophy of the deep muscle of the posterior bladder neck, thereby elevating it and creating a posterior lip. The functional significance of these observations is unknown. Therefore, the ultrasound classification within Type 2 was made flexible to accommodate investigation of these issues (see Fig. 19 and Box 3).

Finally, what constitutes enough tissue between the urethra and the ejaculatory ducts to indicate significant retrourethral (median lobe) hyperplasia? The problem is amplified because there is no noticeable boundary between the periurethral glandular zone and CZ as visualized on TRUS. The ejaculatory ducts (which usually traverse the CZ) provide the only observable landmark. There is no good solution for this dilemma. For the purposes of this ultrasound classification, some observable enlargement extending into the posterior bladder neck area must arbitrarily be required. The most common subtype of retrourethral hyperplasia is

Box 3: Ultrasound classification of benign prostatic hyperplasia

Type 0: Equal to or less than 25 cm³ showing little or no zonal enlargements (Fig. 21)
Type 1: Bilateral TZ (lateral lobe) enlargement (Fig. 22) = 35%
Type 2: Retrourethral (median) enlargement (Figs. 19 and 23) = 10%

> 2a: Mild enlargement without herniation through bladder neck or trigonal elevation
> 2b: Greater enlargement, elevation of the trigone without adenoma herniation through bladder neck and without "trapping" of adenoma or anterior displacement of urethra
> 2c: Enlargement, elevation of trigone without herniation through bladder neck but with "trapping" of adenoma with or without anterior displacement of urethra
> 2d: Greater enlargement with herniation of adenoma through bladder neck and further elevation of trigone
> 2e: Mild enlargement without herniation, stimulating muscular hypertrophy and producing a prominent posterior bladder "lip" (prominent lip must be distinguished from bladder-sphincter dyssynergia unrelated to BPH)

Type 3: Bilateral and retrourethral enlargement (Fig. 24) = 46%
Type 4: Pedunculated (Fig. 25)
Type 5: Bilateral and pedunculated (Fig. 26)
Type 6: Subtrigonal (Fig. 27)
Type 7: Other combinations

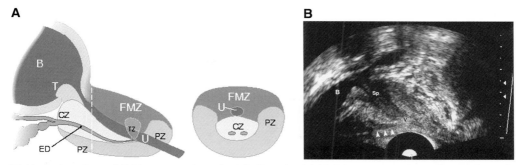

Fig. 21. Normal anatomy. (*A*) Diagrammatic sagittal (*left*) and axial (*right*) representations of normal zonal anatomy before BPH. Dashed line indicates axial plane depicted. B, bladder, ED, ejaculatory duct; FMZ, fibromuscular zone; T, trigone; U, urethra. (*B*) Sagittal TRUS image showing normal ultrasound anatomy. Ejaculatory ducts are indicated by arrowheads. B, bladder; Sp, preprostatic sphincter; V, verumontanum.

Type 2c, whether seen independently or as part of Types 3 or 7 BPH.

After modifying Randall's classification and applying it to 100 consecutive patients evaluated with TRUS, the author found that ultrasound Types 1 and 3 predominated (see Box 3). Examples of the proposed ultrasound classification of BPH are shown in Figs. 21–27.

Notable differences between Randall's cohort and the author's were the preponderance of pedunculated enlargements reported in the former compared with what is detected with TRUS and reported by endoscopists at the author's institution. Randall described most of these as small but "frequently obstructive out of proportion to their size due to their strategic position." In the author's series, solitary pedunculated nodules or pedunculated masses in association with lateral lobe hyperplasia were distinctly unusual. Most median lobe enlargements were of the deep PUG type and occurred in about the same proportion as seen by Randall. In the current series, bilateral lateral lobe

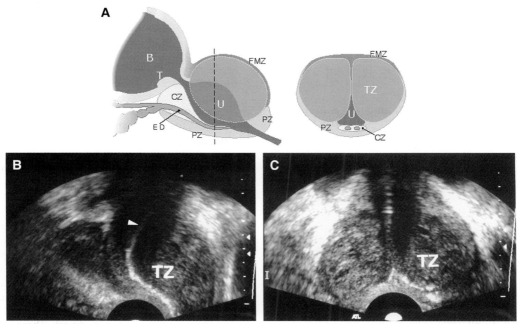

Fig. 22. Ultrasound Type 1 BPH (bilateral TZ). (*A*) Diagrammatic sagittal (*left*) and axial (*right*) views. Note bilateral compression and distortion of urethra (U) into elongated AP slit and compression of overlying CZ and PZ by the enlarged TZ. Dashed line indicates axial plane. B, bladder; ED, ejaculatory duct; FMZ, fibromuscular zone; T, trigone. (*B,C*) TRUS Type 1 BPH in sagittal (*B*) and axial (*C*) views. The course of the urethra is easily identified in the sagittal view by extensive submucosal urethral calcification (*arrowhead*). The enlargement of the TZ crosses the midline enough to displace the urethra posteriorly.

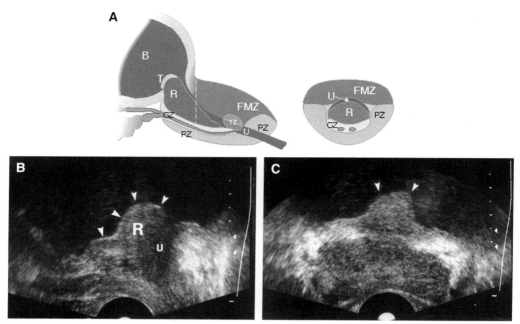

Fig. 23. Ultrasound Type 2 BPH (solitary retrourethral). (*A*) Diagrammatic sagittal (*left*) and axial (*right*) illustrations. Note that the growth is extravesical and elevating the entire bladder trigone. There is compression of the CZ. With greater enlargement, there would be anterior displacement of the urethra (U). Dashed line indicates axial plane. B, bladder; FMZ, fibromuscular zone; R, retrourethral (median) lobe; T, trigone. (*B,C*) TRUS Type 2c BPH sagittal (*B*) and axial (*C*) views. Note extralumenal elevation of bladder trigone (*arrowheads*).

hyperplasia with or without retrourethral enlargement dominated.

Some of the difference in frequency of reported types between the author's study and Randall's [46] is likely due to sampling bias and techniques. Randall's [46] patients were a municipal general hospital population from a poor socioeconomic setting. A large percentage was black (35%) and young (average age at death was 42 years compared with 54 years for whites). It has been shown that hyperplasia occurs first in the PUG before affecting the TZ [11]. Randall [46] noted that pedunculated enlargement (hyperplasia of the superficial PUG) was more common in younger men. Although the average age of the author's patients who had pedunculated enlargement was not significantly different from that of patients who had other types of BPH, the author cannot discount the effect of more advanced age, far fewer African Americans, and a totally different socioeconomic status on the apparent predominance of other patterns in the author's series. Another possible explanation for differences in frequencies of enlargement patterns is the difficulty of clearly making the diagnosis of pedunculated hyperplasia, which rests on being able to demonstrate the position of the polypoid mass inside the bladder or bladder neck (overlying the trigone). Only larger pedunculated adenomas are resolved with TRUS (Fig. 28). Small ones, especially

those within the usually coapted urethral walls, are difficult to visualize without invasive studies. Randall [46] described subtrigonal adenomatous tissue as a rare finding (0.01%), whereas the author saw subtrigonal adenomas more frequently. This difference may also relate to demographics of the current group, but the area posterior to the bladder neck and posterior bladder wall is usually well visualized on the longitudinal TRUS, increasing the probability of detection. Because this type of BPH has not been previously diagnosed in life, there are no studies of the effects of subtrigonal hyperplasia on function. Isolated subtrigonal hyperplasia, because of its location, is unlikely to produce obstructive symptoms unless extensive.

Randall [46] discussed, at length, the diagnosis of "fibrous median bar," pointing out that this had nothing to do with BPH. Pathologically, prominent upper posterior fibrous bars were due to extensive scarring from chronic indolent infection. In his population of patients, it was always due to tuberculosis or syphilis and could be recognized by the associated upward retraction of the verumontanum almost to the undersurface of the bar. Although cystoscopists casually use the term *median bar* with regularity, there are no documented cases of fibrous median bars in the author's series.

There are some other observations that can be made with TRUS that raise clinical and research

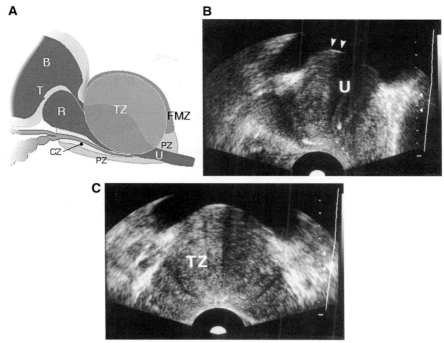

Fig. 24. Ultrasound Type 3 BPH (bilateral and retrourethral). (*A*) Diagrammatic sagittal illustration. B, bladder; FMZ, fibromuscular zone; R, retrourethral (median) lobe; T, trigone; U, urethra. (*B,C*) TRUS ultrasound Type 3 BPH sagittal (*B*) and axial (*C*) views demonstrating enlargement of the retrourethral tissue displacing the urethral structures (U) more vertically and anterior. Note the strong reflection off the elevated thick trigone (*arrowheads*).

questions. For example, what is the relationship between thinning of the PZ and herniation of the TZ through the bladder neck to symptoms and urodynamic measures of obstruction? Which is more symptomatic and clinically serious, an enlarging TZ adenoma "trapped" below the bladder neck and compressing the PZ or the one bulging through the bladder neck into the bladder (see Figs. 16 and 17)? What is the functional significance of the different subtypes of periurethral (median lobe)

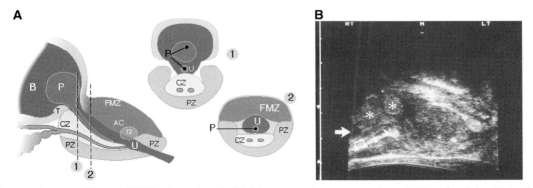

Fig. 25. Ultrasound Type 4 BPH (pedunculated). (*A*) Diagrammatic representation of Albarrán's lobe. Note that the hyperplasia that arises from the superficial submucosal PUG grows entirely within the urethral lumen and migrates on a long pedicle along the path of least resistance into the bladder (B) where it lies anterior to the trigone (T). It is covered only by a thin uroepithelial lining. (See Fig. 18 *C, D*). It does not compress prostatic tissues but obstructs the bladder neck by a ball-valve mechanism. Dashed lines and numbers indicated axial planes. AC, anterior commissure in midline; AFM, anterior fibromuscular zone; FMZ, fibromuscular zone; P, pedunculated adenoma; U, urethra. (*B*) Sagittal view TRUS Type 4 BPH. Rare case of two pedunculated intralumenal adenomas (*asterisks*) anterior to the trigone (*arrowheads*) within the bladder neck and proximal urethra. The arrow points to the acute angle formed by the polyp and trigone.

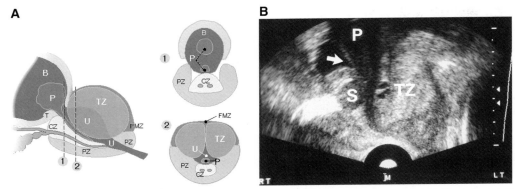

Fig. 26. Ultrasound Type 5 BPH (bilateral and pedunculated). (*A*) Diagrammatic sagittal (*left*) and axial (*right*) illustrations. Note that the TZs are enlarged. The pedunculated tissue protrudes through the bladder neck projecting above the bladder trigone. Dashed lines and numbers indicate axial planes. B, bladder; FMZ, fibromuscular zone; P, pedunculated adenoma; T, trigone; U, urethra. (*B*) Sagittal TRUS image showing Type 5 BPH. Note the relationship of the pedunculated mass projecting above the bladder neck and anterior to the bladder trigone (*arrow*). P, pedunculated (Albarrán's) lobe; S, subtrigonal hyperplasia (technically making this a Type 7).

hyperplasia? When we see no significant prostatic enlargement or a normal sized prostate with a prominent muscular vesicourethral sphincter in a patient with LUTS, may we presume that no obstruction exists or that the dominant mechanism of obstruction is dynamic rather than static and thus more amenable to treatment with α_1-blocking agents? When we see marked TZ or retrourethral (median lobe) hyperplasia, may we presume that the static forces dominate, making it sensible to treat first with 5α-reductase inhibitors? Is there any correlation at all between qualitative sonographic appearance of the prostate gland and the mechanisms producing LUTS or BPO? Could random TRUS-guided biopsy clarify stromal/epithelial ratio and assist in selecting more specific medical management at the onset of therapy? The answers

to these and other questions could be better pursued if we had a reference system to catalog different patterns and distributions of BPH so that they may be individually indexed and compared with symptoms and urodynamic measurements of bladder function and BOO.

Various treatments currently exist for LUTS and particularly for patients diagnosed with BPH. These treatments include the traditional surgical ones (open surgery and TURP), minimally invasive surgery, and pharmacotherapy. There is an ethical and economic imperative to move as directly as possible to the treatment most likely to be effective for the patient. TRUS has the potential to help in this process [7].

Until now, treatment strategies for LUTS have been tested on patient groups among whom there

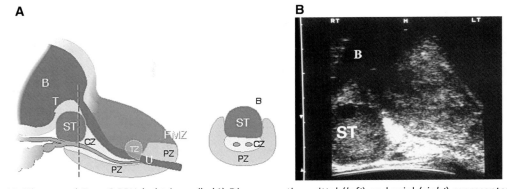

Fig. 27. Ultrasound Type 6 BPH (subtrigonal). (*A*) Diagrammatic sagittal (*left*) and axial (*right*) representations. Note that the hyperplastic tissue is high and "disembodied" from the usual distributions of the median lobe that commonly begin near the verumontanum and extend in continuity upward into the region of the bladder neck (see **Fig. 23**). Dashed line indicates axial plane. B, bladder; FMZ, fibromuscular zone; ST, subtrigonal hyperplasia; T, trigone; U, urethra. (*B*) Sagittal view TRUS image showing Type 6 BPH. Subtrigonal hyperplasia (ST) cannot be appreciated on cystoscopy and rarely, by itself, has a significant obstructive effect because it is outside the prostatic capsule and bladder (B).

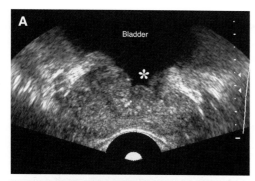

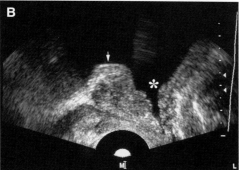

Fig. 28. Postoperative changes of TURP. (*A*) Axial TRUS view demonstrating the generous TURP defect (*asterisk*). (*B*) Sagittal TRUS view demonstrating the generous TURP defect (*asterisk*). Note the strong echo of the bladder trigone (*arrow*).

has been little distinction in type of hyperplasia: strategy A is compared with strategy B or placebo. Until now, global measures of therapeutic outcome and conclusions have been made as though the experimental group was affected by only one disease. The treatment does or does not work compared with placebo or TURP. The only way such studies are ordinarily stratified is by prostatic volume [48]. The First International Consultation of BPH recommended "future studies should seek determinants, or predictors of BPH parameters," calling for "larger studies with adequate power for subgroup analysis" [49].

The proposed preliminary ultrasound classification of BPH is presented as a work in progress [50]. Much research is necessary to establish its usefulness, beginning with a prospective correlative study with cystoscopy involving urologists thoroughly familiar with the classifications. Validation of the system in the hands of other ultrasound interpreters is also recommended. Because the author's preliminary study involved decisions by a single experienced observer only, the general applicability of this classification system must be tested to determine interobserver reliability. Modifications are expected. Meanwhile, this classification

is presented in the hope that it may ultimately be used to stratify BPH for diagnostic and therapeutic research and remind us that we are dealing with a complex anatomic and physiologic disorder not likely to reveal its secrets as currently being studied.

The appearance of BPH using MR imaging and MR spectroscopy has been recently reviewed [51].

Postoperative changes

The most common surgical treatment for BPH is TURP. This endoscopic-guided procedure uses a hot cutting wire. The heat of the wire tends to cauterize the base of the tissue defect to limit bleeding. The level of the resection is mainly above the verumontanum to preclude trauma to and scarring of the openings of the ejaculatory ducts. As each chip of tissue is resected, it is placed into the bladder, allowing an accumulation that is periodically flushed out with fluid. The resectionist continues to remove tissue until the stretched smooth muscle pseudocapsule (surgical capsule) is identified by its muscle fibers. Progressively deep resection of TZ tissue is not very precise, however, and commonly the

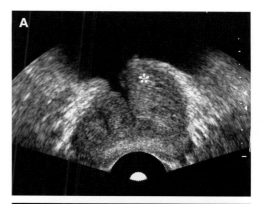

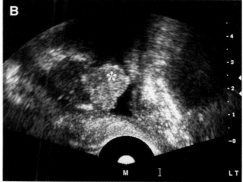

Fig. 29. Hyperplastic regrowth of TZ tissue. Axial TRUS view (*A*) and sagittal TRUS view (*B*) showing asymmetric regrowth of the TZ on the left side (*asterisk*) following TURP. The triangular TURP defect is clear on the sagittal projection.

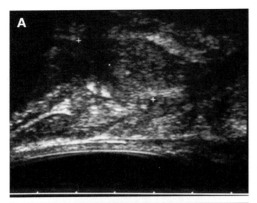

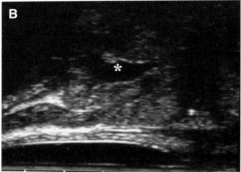

Fig. 30. (*A*) Preoperative appearance of mild TZ BPH. (*B*) Three-month postoperative changes following TUEVP. A surgical defect is seen in the prostate superior to the verumontanum (*asterisk*). This appearance is similar to those following TURP, laser, and other minimally invasive therapies.

surgical capsule is pierced and some PZ tissue removed. Occasionally, when the PZ is thinned and compressed by the large expansile TZ, the "true" capsule is breached and some periprostatic fat can be seen. The resultant TURP defect seen on imaging is a central prostatic cavity of variable volume and shape above the verumontanum, often including a widened bladder neck (see Fig. 28A). The large defect in the operative field while it is distended with fluids is significantly smaller when seen on postoperative imaging in the undistended state but will distend further with urine flow (see Fig. 28B). The boundaries of the prostatic defect may appear shaggy at first until re-epithelialization occurs. Significant TZ tissue may remain in the periphery of the defect, which does not usually affect functional results unless there is significant later regrowth (Fig. 29).

Similarly, some surgeons use a "roller ball" head as a substitute for the cutting wire [52]. Because its surface area is greater than the cutting wire, a much higher temperature can be used, resulting in almost complete vaporization of TZ tissue, further limiting bleeding and recovery time. Vaporization with the roller ball and laser surgery in various

forms also produce a typical TURP-appearing defect on subsequent imaging studies (Fig. 30). More recent minimally invasive techniques tend to produce less cavitation defects but overall decreased volume of the subepithelial hyperplastic–ablated TZ tissue.

Prostatic urethral stents have been inserted for short-term relief of obstruction at the level of the prostate and bladder neck [53]. Careful documentation of stent positioning using TRUS or radiography is advisable to preclude the superior tip resting above the bladder neck where precipitation of calcium may cause permanent encrustation, making removal difficult and predisposing to bladder infection and stones.

Acknowledgments

I wish to express my deepest thanks to Ann Toobin Wasserman for her manuscript reviews, suggestions, and other innumerable assistances for this article and all previous articles and poster presentations leading up to this article.

References

[1] Chute CG, Panser LA, et al. Prevalence of prostatism: a population based survey of urinary symptoms. J Urol 1993;150:85.

[2] Nakajima H. In: Denis L, Griffiths K, Khoury S, et al, editors. 4th International Consultation on Benign Prostatic Hyperplasia, Paris, July 2–5, 1997. Plymoth, UK: Plymbridge Distributors Ltd.; 1998. p. 20.

[3] Berry SJ, Coffey DS, Walsh PC, et al. The development of human benign prostatic hyperplasia with age. J Urol 1984;132:474–9.

[4] Roehrborn CG, McConnell JD. Etiology, pathophysiology, epidemiology and natural history of benign prostatic hyperplasia. In: Walsh PC, Retik AB, Vaughn EB Jr, et al, editors. Campbell's urology. 8th edition. Philadelphia: WB Saunders Co.; 2002. p. 38, 1297–330.

[5] Abrams P. New words for old: lower urinary tract symptoms for "prostatism.". BMJ 1994;308:929–30.

[6] Koyanagi T, Artibani W, Correa R, et al. Initial diagnostic evaluation of men with lower urinary tract symptoms. In: Denis L, Griffiths K, Khoury S, et al, editors. 4th International Consultation on Benign Prostatic Hyperplasia, Paris, July 2–5, 1997. Plymoth, UK: Plymbridge Distributors Ltd.; 1998. p. 183–4.

[7] AUA Practice Guidelines Committee. AUA guideline on management of benign prostatic hyperplasia. Chapter 1: diagnosis and treatment recommendations. J Urol 2003;170:530–47.

[8] Ohe H, Ohnishi K, Watanabe H, et al. Accuracy of digital palpation for size assessment of the prostate evaluated by transrectal ultrasound. Tohoku J Exp Med 1988;154:323–8.

[9] McNeal J. The prostate and prostatic urethra: a morphologic synthesis. J Urol 1972;107: 1008–15.

[10] McNeal JE. Pathology of benign prostatic hyperplasia. Urol Clin North Am 1990;17:477–86.

[11] McNeal JE. Origin and evolution of benign prostatic enlargement. Invest Urol 1978;15:340–5.

[12] McNeal JE. Normal histology of the prostate. Am J Surg Path 1988;12:619–33.

[13] Blacklock NJ. Surgical anatomy of the prostate. In: Williams DI, Chisholm GD, editors. Scientific foundations of urology. Chicago: William Heinemann Medical Books Ltd., Year Book Medical Publishers; 1976. p. 473–85.

[14] Tanagho EA. Postprostatectomy incontinence: urodynamic evaluation. In: Hinman F Jr, editor. Benign prostatic hypertrophy. New York: Springer-Verlag; 1983. p. 985–96.

[15] Hutch JA, Rambo ON Jr. A study of the anatomy of the prostate, prostatic urethra and the urinary sphincter system. J Urol 1970;104:443–52.

[16] Turner-Warwick R. Sphincter mechanisms: their relation to prostatic enlargement and its treatment. In: Hinman F Jr, editor. Benign prostatic hypertrophy. New York: Springer-Verlag; 1983. p. 809–28.

[17] Oelrich TM. The urethral sphincter muscle in the male. Am J Anat 1980;158:229–46.

[18] Sattar AA, Noel J-C, Vanderhaeghen J-J, et al. Prostate capsule: computerized morphometric analysis of its components. Urology 1995;46: 178–81.

[19] Griffiths K, Cockett ATK, Coffey D, et al. Regulation of prostatic growth. In: Denis L, Griffiths K, Khoury S, et al O, editors. 4th International Consultation on Benign Prostatic Hyperplasia, Paris July 2–5, 1997. Plymoth, UK: Plymbridge Distributors Ltd.; 1998. p. 83–128.

[20] Taoka R, Tsukuda F, Ishikawa M, et al. Association of prostatic inflammation with down-regulation of macrophage inhibitory cytokine-1 gene in symptomatic benign prostatic hyperplasia. J Urol 2004;171:2330–5.

[21] Price H, McNeal JE, Stamey TA. Evolving patterns of tissue composition in benign prostatic hyperplasia as a function of specimen size. Hum Pathol 1990;21:578–85.

[22] Shapiro E, Hartanto V, Lepor H. The response to alpha blockade in benign prostatic hyperplasia is related to the percent area density of prostate smooth muscle. Prostate 1992;21:297–307.

[23] Robert M, Costa P, Bressolle F, et al. Percentage area of epithelial and mesenchymal components in benign prostatic hyperplasia: comparison of results between single biopsy, multiple biopsies, and multiple tissue specimens. Br J Urol 1995; 75:317–24.

[24] Deering RE, Bigler SA, King J, et al. Morphometric quantitation of stroma in human benign prostatic hyperplasia. Urology 1994;44:64–70.

[25] Ishigooka M, Haymi S, Hashimoto T, et al. Relative and total volume of histological components in benign prostatic hyperplasia: relationships between histological components and clinical findings. Prostate 1996;29:77–82.

[26] Marks LS, Treiger B, Dorey FJ, et al. Morphology of the prostate: distribution of tissue components in hyperplastic glands. Urology 1996;44: 486–92.

[27] Zlotta AR, Sattar AA, Wespes E, et al. Is one single prostate biopsy helpful for choosing a medical treatment of benign prostatic hyperplasia? A quantitative computerized morphometric study. Urology 1996;47:329–34.

[28] Leissner K-H, Tisell L-E. The weight of the human prostate. Scand J Urol Nephrol 1979;13: 137–42.

[29] Greene DR, Egawa S, Hellerstein DK, et al. Sonographic measurements of transition zone of prostate in men with and without benign prostatic hyperplasia. Urology 1990;36:293–9.

[30] Jakobsen H, Torp-Pedersen S, Juul N. Ultrasonic evaluation of age-related human prostatic growth and development of benign prostatic hyperplasia. Scand J Urol Nephrol Suppl 1988; 107:26–31.

[31] Aarnink RG, de la Rosette JJMCH, Huynen AL, et al. Standardized assessment to enhance the diagnostic value of prostate volume; part I: morphometry in patients with lower urinary tract symptoms. Prostate 1996;29:317–26.

[32] Tang J, Li X, Wang N, et al. Correlation between hypoechoic nodules on ultrasonography and benign hyperplasia in the prostatic outer gland. J Ultrasound Med 2005;24:483–8.

[33] Hasegawa Y, Sakamoto N, Gotoh K. Relationship of ultrasonic and histologic findings in benign prostatic hyperplasia. Prostate 1996;28: 111–6.

[34] Kaplan SA, Te AE, Pressler LB, et al. Transition zone index as a method of assessing benign prostatic hyperplasia: correlation with symptoms, urine flow and detrusor pressure. J Urol 1995;154:1764–9.

[35] Kojima M, Ochiai A, Naya Y, et al. Correlation of presumed circle area ratio with infravesical obstruction in men with lower urinary tract symptoms. Urology 1997;50:548–55.

[36] Tewari A, Shinohara K, Narayan P. Transition zone volume and transition zone ratio: predictor of uroflow response to finasteride therapy in benign prostatic hyperplasia patients. Urology 1995;45:258–64.

[37] Littrup PJ, Williams CH, Egglin TK, et al. Determination of prostate volume with transrectal ultrasonography for cancer screening. Radiology 1991;179:49–53.

[38] Bangma CH, Niemer AQHJ, Grobbee DE, et al. Transrectal ultrasonic volumetry of the prostate: in vivo comparison of different methods. Prostate 1996;28:107–10.

[39] Terris MK, Stamey TA. Determination of prostate volume by transrectal ultrasound. J Urol 1991; 145:984–7.

[40] Roehborn CG, McConnell JD. Etiology, patho-physiology, epidemiology and natural history of benign prostatic hyperplasia. In: Walsh PC, Retik AB, Vaughn ED Jr, et al, editors. Campbell's urology. 8th edition. Philadelphia: WB Saunders Co.; 2002. p. 1297–330.

[41] Orandi A. Transurethral incision of prostate (TUIP) 646 cases in 15 years—a chronological appraisal. Br J Urol 1985;57:703–7.

[42] Riehmann M, Knes JM, Heisey D, et al. Transurethral resection versus incision of the prostate: a randomized, prospective study. Urology 1995; 45:768–75.

[43] Kabalin JN. Laser prostatectomy performed with a right angle firing neodymium: YAG laser fiber at 40 watts power setting. J Urol 1993;150: 90–5.

[44] Boyle P, Gould AL, Roehborn CG. Prostate volume predicts outcome of treatment of benign prostatic hyperplasia with finasteride: meta-analysis of randomized clinical trials. Urology 1996;48:398–405.

[45] Wasserman NF. Imaging benign prostatic hyperplasia. Contemporary Radiology 1999;11: 81–94.

[46] Randall A. Surgical pathology of prostatic obstructions. Baltimore (MD): Williams & Wilkins; 1931.

[47] Randall A, Hinman F Jr. Surgical anatomy of the prostatic lobes. In: Hinman F Jr, editor. Benign prostatic hypertrophy. New York: Springer-Verlag; 1983. p. 672–7.

[48] Lepor H, Williford WO, Barry MJ, et al. The efficiency of terazosin, finasteride or both in benign prostatic hyperplasia. N Engl J Med 1996;335: 533–9.

[49] Barry MJ, Beckley S, Boyle P, et al. Importance of understanding the epidemiology and natural history of BPH. In: Cockett ATK, Aso Y, Chatelain C, et al, editors. Proceedings of the International consultation on benign prostatic hyperplasia (BPH). Paris: Scientific Communications International Ltd.; 1991. p. 37.

[50] Wasserman NF. Distribution patterns of benign prostatic hyperplasia: importance and preliminary ultrasound classification. Poster presentation at the 88th Scientific Assembly and Annual Meeting of the Radiological Society of North America. Chicago, November 30–December 6, 2002.

[51] Grossfeld GD, Coakley FV. Benign prostatic hyperplasia: clinical overview and value of diagnostic imaging. Radiol Clin North Am 2000;38:31–47.

[52] Kupeli S, Soygur T, Yilmaz E, et al. Combined transurethral resection and vaporization of the prostate using newly designed electrode: a promising treatment alternative for benign prostatic hyperplasia. J Endourol 1999;13:225–8.

[53] Djavan B, Fakhari M, Shariat S, et al. A novel intraurethral prostatic bridge catheter for prevention of temporary prostatic obstruction following high-energy transurethral microwave thermotherapy in patients with benign prostatic hyperplasia. J Urol 1999;161:144–51.

RADIOLOGIC
CLINICS
OF NORTH AMERICA

Radiol Clin N Am 44 (2006) 711–722

Prostate Cancer Imaging—What the Urologic Oncologist Needs to Know

Robert Ross, MD[a,b,*], Mukesh Harisinghani, MD[b]

- Prostate cancer imaging
- Disease state 1: patients who do not have a prostate cancer diagnosis
  Ultrasound techniques
  Recommendations
- Disease state 2: patients who have clinically localized prostate cancer
  MR imaging to differentiate T2 from T3 disease
  The use of lymphtrophic nanoparticle MR imaging to identify lymph node involvement
  The use of bone scintigraphy to identify bone metastases

Use of 2-deoxy-2-[^{18}F]fluoro-D-glucose positron emission tomography
Recommendations
- Disease state 3: rising prostate-specific antigen
  Identification of local recurrence using MR imaging
  Novel radiolabeled antibody techniques
  Bone scintigraphy
  Use of 2-deoxy-2-[^{18}F]fluoro-D-glucose positron emission tomography
  Recommendations
- Summary
- References

Prostate cancer is the most commonly diagnosed malignancy and the second most common cause of cancer death of men in the United States [1]. Appropriate imaging is a crucial component of staging and therapy application. Yet, the optimal imaging algorithm in prostate cancer is constantly changing. The goal of this review is to delineate the appropriate use of imaging modalities such as bone scanning (BS), helical CT scanning, ultrasound (US), positron emission tomography (PET), and MR imaging.

Scher and Heller [2] recently described a prostate cancer organizational schema that divides the possible patient presentations into several disease states: no cancer diagnosis, clinically localized disease, rising prostate-specific antigen (PSA) levels, and clinical metastases (noncastrate and castrate). This article focuses on the disease states of no cancer diagnosis, clinically localized disease, and rising PSA because these states are most germane to the urologic oncologist. Within each of these disease states, the most relevant imaging modalities are considered.

Prostate cancer imaging

Several aspects of prostate cancer biology have posed challenges to the development of imaging techniques. The soft tissue planes of the prostate are difficult to clearly resolve on conventional

[a] Dana 1230, Dana Farber Cancer Institute, 44 Binney Street, Boston, MA 0211, USA
[b] Center for Molecular Imaging Research, Massachusetts General Hospital, Charlestown Navy Yard, 149 13th Street, Room 5406, Charlestown, MA 02129-2060, USA
* Corresponding author. Dana 1230, Dana Farber Cancer Institute, 44 Binney Street, Boston, MA 0211, USA.
E-mail address: rwross@partners.org (R. Ross).

0033-8389/06/$ – see front matter © 2006 Elsevier Inc. All rights reserved.
radiologic.theclinics.com

doi:10.1016/j.rcl.2006.07.002

imaging, and benign prostatic hypertrophy is hard to distinguish from prostate cancer. The low proliferation rate of early prostate cancer results in decreased uptake of some contrast agents, and its propensity to spread to bone makes assessment of treatment response difficult. Moreover, the clinical trial design of many imaging modalities in prostate cancer has often considered patients who have a wide range of disease states, making it hard to draw conclusions about the utility of the modalities in specific clinical situations [2,3]. Despite these challenges, there is a role for several imaging techniques in prostate cancer, including US, MR imaging, BS, and PET (Table 1). Table 2 provides a summary of novel types of imaging that have promise in prostate cancer.

Disease state 1: patients who do not have a prostate cancer diagnosis

This disease state consists of men who do not have a tissue (biopsy) diagnosis but have a high clinical suspicion due to a positive digital rectal examination or a high or rapidly rising PSA. Occasionally, for men who initially present with symptoms of locally advanced or metastatic disease (bone pain, weight loss, pelvic pain), local prostate imaging may be less appropriate. With the advent of PSA screening protocols, there has been a significant stage migration in newly diagnosed prostate cancer [4]. Most cancers are less extensive at presentation, making visualization difficult. The imaging technique with the most utility in this situation is US,

although recent data regarding MR spectroscopy have been encouraging.

Ultrasound techniques

Transrectal ultrasonography (TRUS) produces high-resolution, operator-dependent axial, sagittal, and oblique images of the prostate using an endorectal high-frequency (7.5 MHz) transducer, typically using gray-scale alone. It is unfortunate that up to 40% of lesions may be isoechoic and undetectable [5]. TRUS alone has poor test characteristics for the diagnosis of prostate cancer, with a positive predictive value of 52.7%, a negative predictive value of 72%, and an accuracy of 67% in modern series [6]. In combination with a set of six biopsy cores (sextant biopsy), false-negative rates still approach 34%. Common strategies to decrease false-negative rates include increasing biopsy number (from 12 to as high as 45 in a saturation biopsy approach) [7,8] and lateral and anterior biopsies [9,10].

Newer US techniques include color Doppler, power Doppler, and contrast agents [10]. Color and power Doppler use reflected sound waves to evaluate blood flow through local vessels (power Doppler may be more sensitive to smaller vessels) [11]. Microbubble contrast agents have recently been reported to improve detection of tumor vascularity [12,13]. Because higher blood flow is often associated with tumor, these techniques help to "target" prostate biopsies. Even with these improvements, the positive and negative predictive values of biopsies targeted by a power Doppler US approach are still suboptimal [6,14]. In two studies, contrast-enhanced US had a similar detection rate to

Table 1: **Imaging techniques in prostate cancer**

Imaging modality	Advantages	Disadvantages	Newer techniques
US	Less expensive; quick	Operator dependent; poor sensitivity and specificity	Contrast-enhanced US
MR imaging	High soft tissue resolution	Expensive; quality between sites varies; discomfort associated with an endorectal coil	MRS LNMR imaging DCE MR imaging
BS	High sensitivity for bone metastases	Poor specificity, especially early in disease; planar images	SPECT BS
PET	Whole-body tomography images; ability to measure cellular processes	Expensive; problems with radiotracer elimination through the urinary system	PET/CT
Radiolabeled antibody	Highly specific antibody	Planar images hard to interpret	Coregistration with CT/ MR imaging

Abbreviations: DCE, dynamic contrast-enhanced; LNMR imaging, lymphtrophic nanoparticle MR imaging; MRS, MR spectroscopy; SPECT, Single-photon emission tomography.

Table 2:   **Summary of novel imaging techniques in prostate cancer**

Modality	Novel technique	Advantages	Disadvantages
US	Contrast-enhanced US	Higher sensitivity for vascular lesions; fewer biopsies needed	Requires unapproved contrast agent; false positives associated with prostatitis
MR imaging	LNMR imaging	Improved lymph node staging	Requires unapproved contrast agent; clinical data limited to few patients
	MRS	Differentiation between prostate cancer and normal prostate or necrotic tissue	Published data only from a few sites; hemorrhage artifact; difficulty with TZ cancers
	DCE-MR imaging	Higher sensitivity for vascular lesions	Requires contrast agent; hemorrhage artifacts; clinical data limited to few patients
SPECT	SPECT BS	Higher specificity at differentiating prostate metastases from arthritis	Little data in prostate cancer; only a limited skeletal area can be imaged in a reasonable time
PET	Novel radioligands	Potential detection of early lesions; ability to follow treatment-related changes	Difficulties with normal ligand excretion (FDG); need for an on-site cyclotron (11-carbon compounds)

Abbreviations: DCE, dynamic contrast-enhanced; FDG, 2-deoxy-2-[18F] fluoro-D-glucose; LNMR imaging, lymphtrophic nanoparticle MR imaging; MRS, MR spectroscopy; SPECT, Single-photon emission tomography; TZ, transitional zone.

standard gray-scale US but allowed for fewer biopsies (contrast-enhanced US was three times more likely to detect prostate cancer on a per-biopsy basis) [12,15]. Limitations to these novel US approaches include the hypervascularity of benign prostatic hypertrophy (making transitional zone cancers hard to detect), false positives associated with prostatitis, and the fact that lower Gleason score cancers are less vascular (which may be of little relevance because Gleason grade is significantly associated with risk of prostate cancer–specific death [16]).

Recommendations

Overall, in patients who do not have a diagnosis of prostate cancer, US remains the mainstay of prostate cancer detection. As contrast-enhanced US techniques become more widely used, this technique may be able to provide similar information with fewer biopsies. Men who have a rising PSA but multiple negative biopsies remain a clinical conundrum but represent a good population for the study of new imaging modalities in this disease state (eg, a recent study has demonstrated that MR spectroscopy might be useful in this situation [17]).

Disease state 2: patients who have clinically localized prostate cancer

Imaging in the clinically localized disease state can provide useful information. Differentiating between T3 disease (prostate cancer that has spread outside the prostatic capsule) and T2 disease (prostate cancer confined within the capsule) is critical because it often drives the decision to use radiation therapy as opposed to radical prostatectomy. Moreover, preoperative (or preradiotherapy) identification of involved lymph nodes is of benefit in deciding whether a localized treatment modality is warranted. One of the few places where early androgen deprivation therapy has been shown to improve survival is in patients who have positive lymph nodes after radical prostatectomy [18]. Yet, commonly used imaging approaches in this disease state (pelvic CT, body-coil MR imaging, and

TRUS) are limited by lack of sensitivity in identifying T3 disease and lymph node involvement [1,19–23].

MR imaging to differentiate T2 from T3 disease

The value of non–contrast-enhanced MR imaging in this disease state is in its ability to differentiate T2 from T3 disease (Fig. 1). This differentiation is best achieved using an endorectal coil, although controversy still exists as to whether endorectal coil MR imaging (erMR imaging) provides improved sensitivity compared with MR imaging with a pelvic coil. A recent meta-analysis found that erMR imaging had a combined sensitivity and specificity of 71% at distinguishing T2 from T3 disease [24]; however, these numbers are inflated because of the promising results from smaller, single-center studies. A large multi-institutional study found an accuracy of erMR imaging of only 54% [25].

Several methods are currently used to improve these test characteristics. The first is patient selection: although erMR imaging has no role in low-risk, clinically localized disease, it may provide some useful information in clinically localized but higher-risk disease [1,26–30]. No study has shown, however, that changing management strategies based on erMR imaging results improves patient outcomes.

The second method used to improve erMR imaging at distinguishing T2 from T3 disease is the use of dynamic contrast enhancement and the use of spectroscopy (MR spectroscopy). Dynamic contrast-enhanced (DCE) MR imaging uses the infusion of a macromolecular contrast agent (usually gadolinium) and MR imaging (often with an endorectal coil) to visualize tumor vascularity. Because prostate cancers are usually hypervascular compared with normal prostate, DCE MR imaging may be able to help detect and accurately stage prostate cancer. Several studies have reported on the ability of DCE MR imaging to detect prostate cancer [31–38], and researchers are still trying to identify the best criteria to use to differentiate benign from malignant disease.

Spectroscopy relies on the fact that MR imaging uses a strong magnetic field to force hydrogen protons into uniform spinning and then generates a map of signal intensities by three-dimensional location using radiofrequency pulses and spatially varying magnetic-field gradients. The signals from different hydrogen protons vary slightly according to their molecule, a phenomenon known as chemical shift. MR spectroscopy plots these chemical shifts against spatial localization such that within each voxel, peaks representing the frequency and intensity of various molecules can be traced [39]. Important molecules in prostate cancer MR spectroscopy include choline, creatine, and citrate. Prostate cancer is identifiable by an increased choline-to-citrate ratio [40], which can also be correlated to Gleason grade [41].

Several studies have demonstrated that compared with erMR imaging alone, MR spectroscopy has higher specificity but lower sensitivity [42]. The combination of these modalities can lead to high sensitivity and specificity for peripheral zone tumor localization [43] but is only able to detect tumors greater than 0.5 cm^3 [44]. In one study that evaluated erMR imaging alone and erMR imaging with MR spectroscopy, the accuracy of the diagnosis of extracapsular extension of prostate cancer was improved with MR spectroscopy only in readers who had less experience [45]. The American College of Radiology Imaging Network has undertaken a multi-institutional trial of MR spectroscopy. Higher magnet strength (3 T) may also have a role in improving erMR imaging in general and MR spectroscopy in particular [46].

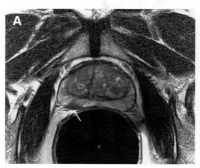 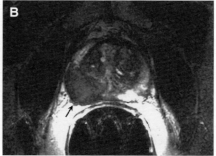

Fig. 1. T2-weighted endorectal coil MR imaging of patients who had prostate cancer. (*A*) Cancer within the right posterior peripheral zone (*arrow*), without evidence of extracapsular extension. (*B*) Prostate cancer in a different patient in the same location, but with extracapsular extension (*arrow*).

The use of lymphtrophic nanoparticle MR imaging to identify lymph node involvement

The use of iron oxide nanoparticles as an MR imaging contrast agent has recently been shown to be useful in improving the sensitivity and specificity of MR imaging in detecting prostate cancer lymph node involvement. These nanoparticles have an iron oxide core, contain a dense packing of dextrans, and are avidly taken up by lymph nodes in animals and humans, where they cause changes in the magnetic properties of the lymph nodes that are detectable by MR imaging (Fig. 2) [47–49].

Harisinghani and colleagues [50] at the Massachusetts General Hospital in the United States and the University Medical Center in the Netherlands performed the most comprehensive analysis of the use of this contrast agent with MR imaging (called lymphtrophic nanoparticle MR imaging [LNMR imaging]) in men who had localized prostate cancer. In this trial of 80 men who had primarily intermediate to high-risk localized prostate cancer, a total of 334 lymph nodes were resected or underwent biopsy. LNMR imaging (performed before surgery) had a positive predictive value of 95% and a negative predictive value of 97.8% in the detection of nodal metastases (significantly better than MR imaging alone using conventional size criteria for the determination of malignancy). LNMR imaging performed well in the setting of nodes that had a short-axis diameter of 5 to 10 mm, but its test characteristics fell off in the 17 nodes in which the diameter was less than 5 mm, with a positive predictive value of only 77.7% in this setting.

Several caveats are important to note. First, this trial was a comparatively small trial that was performed in only two institutions because iron oxide nanoparticle contrast agent is an investigational agent and only available within the context of a clinical trial. Second, LNMR imaging entails two MR

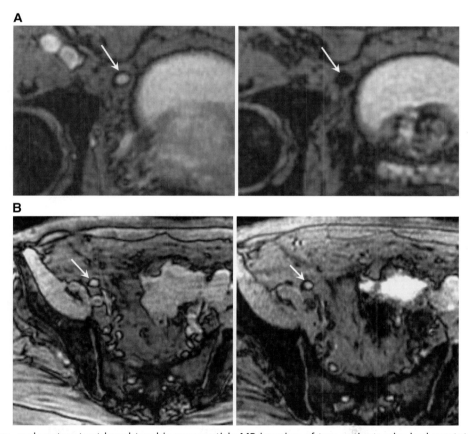

Fig. 2. Pre- and postcontrast lymphtrophic nanoparticle MR imaging of two patients who had prostate cancer. (*A*) Characteristic enhancement of a benign lymph node. The left panel shows the precontrast image; the right panel shows the postcontrast image. Note the homogenous uptake of the iron oxide nanoparticles into the lymph node (*arrow*), causing it to appear dark. (*B*) Characteristic enhancement of a malignant lymph node. The left panel shows the precontrast image; the right panel shows the postcontrast image. Note that the node remains hyperintense (*arrow*), indicating heterogeneous uptake of the iron oxide nanoparticles.

imaging sessions, thus requiring two visits to the MR imaging suite (one before the contrast infusion as a baseline study and another 24 hours after contrast administration), adding to its cost and time consumption. Finally, more research is needed to identify which patient populations would benefit from this procedure and how best to use the information to alter patient care.

The use of bone scintigraphy to identify bone metastases

BS (also known as skeletal scintigraphy) is the most common nuclear medicine test used in prostate cancer. BS can use various radionucleotides including technetium 99m bound to methylene diphosphonate, hydroxymethylene diphosphonate, or dicarboxypropane diphosphonate to visualize increases in osteoblastic activity and vascularization [51]. For the detection of metastases in metastatic prostate cancer, BS has high sensitivity. Yet, one disadvantage of BS is its lack of specificity, especially in men who have only a small number of metastatic sites. The issue of poor specificity of BS is critically important in the clinically localized disease subset of prostate cancer patients for whom detection of metastatic disease is unusual (especially in the PSA era) and would have significant impact on treatment decisions. A recent meta-analysis by Abuzallouf and colleagues [22] considered this issue in detail. These investigators reviewed 23 studies of BS in newly diagnosed prostate cancer and found detection rates of 2.3%, 5.3%, and 16.2% in men who had PSA levels less than 10 ng/mL, 10.1 to 20 ng/mL, and 20.1 to 49 ng/mL, respectively. Detection rates were 6.4% versus 49.5% in men who had clinically localized versus locally advanced disease, and 5.6% versus 29.9% for men who had a Gleason score of 7 or less versus 8 or more. Based on these data, for men in the clinically localized disease setting in the absence of bone symptoms or an elevated alkaline phosphatase, BS should be reserved for patients who have a PSA greater than 20 ng/mL, a Gleason score of 8 or higher, or clinical T3 or T4 disease. Positive BS in men who have clinically localized disease should be confirmed with conventional imaging and, if still questionable, a bone biopsy.

Use of 2-deoxy-2-[^{18}F]fluoro-D-glucose positron emission tomography

PET scans use radiopharmaceuticals that decay by the release of positrons (positively charged electrons) to produce high-resolution, whole-body tomographic images. PET can be combined with CT scanning in one machine to produce high-resolution images [52]. A variety of radioactive substances decay by way of positron emission and can be differentiated by their half-life, including carbon 11 (20 minutes) and fluorine 18 (110 minutes). Radiotracers that have been used in prostate cancer with some success include 2-deoxy-2-[^{18}F]fluoro-D-glucose (FDG), radiolabeled acetate, radiolabeled methionine, radiolabeled choline, and radiolabeled dihydrotestosterone [53–55]. FDG-PET is the technique most developed in prostate cancer. FDG is preferentially taken up by tissues that have increased glycolysis and then phosphorylated by hexokinase and trapped within these cells. Thus, FDG-PET is able to detect the cells that have a hypermetabolic glycoloysis pathway. Its use in prostate cancer is limited by excreted FDG in the ureters and bladder and the observation that many prostate cancers have a relatively low glycolytic rate.

Several investigators have considered FDG-PET radiotracers for staging in localized prostate cancer [56,57]. These data are predominantly negative when considering the primary tumor (except potentially with higher-grade disease) and mixed when considering lymph node involvement (although the lymph node studies are small and uncontrolled) [58–62]. Radiolabeled acetate and choline may be an improvement [56,57,63,64]. In general, the use of PET for the detection of small lymph node involvement is limited by the resolution of this technique (0.5 mm to 1 cm); therefore, its sensitivity is unlikely to approach that of techniques with higher spatial resolution such as MR imaging.

Recommendations

Patients who have clinically localized disease are a heterogeneous group, and the appropriate imaging techniques depend on their risk stratification. Patients at low risk (Gleason score <7, PSA <10 ng/mL, clinically T1c) probably need no imaging at all. Patients at high risk (Gleason score 8–10, PSA >10 ng/mL, or clinical T2c or T3 disease) may benefit from erMR imaging in experienced centers to distinguish T2 from T3 disease and may benefit from BS to evaluate for distant metastases. The data for patients at intermediate risk are not well explored. MR spectroscopy and LNMR imaging may be added to this algorithm as further data are accumulated.

Disease state 3: rising prostate-specific antigen

The rising PSA setting (also called "biochemical recurrence") is one of the most perplexing states of this disease. For most solid tumors, recurrence is heralded by the presence of metastases on imaging tests. PSA testing, however, has created the disease state of biochemical recurrence in which a rising serum PSA indicates disease recurrence, yet no metastases are evident. This disease state can be lengthy, with a time between PSA elevation and development of bone metastases of 8 years in one cohort study of men not treated with androgen deprivation [65]. Even after the development of androgen resistance (defined as a rising PSA while on androgen deprivation therapy), the median time to the development of bone metastasis is still more than 2 years [66]. Moreover, this disease state is common: between 25% and 35% of men treated with local therapy for clinically localized disease eventually experience an asymptomatic biochemical recurrence.

The critical diagnostic dilemma for men who have a rising PSA after local treatment is the differentiation of patients who have local recurrence only (and are therefore candidates for further local therapy) from those who have metastatic spread [67]. Commonly used imaging modalities in this setting include TRUS with biopsy (to confirm local recurrence), pelvic CT scan and erMR imaging (to identify lymph node metastasis and evaluate pelvic bones for evidence of metastatic disease), and BS (to identify metastatic disease). It is unfortunate that these modalities are limited by poor sensitivity, especially in the setting of a low PSA (<5 ng/mL) [68]. Newer modalities for this disease state include indium 111 capromab pendetide (ProstaScint, Cytogen Corp., Princeton, New Jersey), MR spectroscopy, and PET.

Identification of local recurrence using MR imaging

Preliminary data suggest that, in men who have biochemical recurrence after radical prostatectomy, erMR imaging is a useful modality for defining local recurrence. In the most recent study of this modality, Sella and colleagues [69] described a sensitivity of 95% and a specificity of 100% for detecting local recurrence, which was found at the anastomotic site, near retained seminal vesicles, and at the lateral and anterior surgical margins. These data are consistent with early studies using erMR imaging in this disease setting [70].

Identifying local recurrence after radiation therapy with erMR imaging is challenging because treatment-related changes including prostatic shrinkage and diffuse low T2 signal intensity make identification of viable tumor difficult [71–73]. In this setting, MR spectroscopy might prove useful as a method for identifying abnormal metabolism instead of abnormal anatomy. Coakley and colleagues [74] examined 21 patients who had a rising PSA after external beam radiation therapy. All patients also underwent prostate biopsy. Using MR spectroscopy abnormalities on a 1.5-T system (as defined by the number of voxels deemed

suspicious—an elevated choline and an absent citrate peak), the area under the receiver-operating curve was 0.81 for MR spectroscopy, whereas it was only 0.49 to 0.51 with erMR imaging alone. Although these data are preliminary, they suggest that MR spectroscopy is an imaging modality with reasonable test characteristics for patients who have biochemical relapse after external beam radiation.

Novel radiolabeled antibody techniques

Indium 111 capromab pendetide is a radiolabeled murine monoclonal immunoglobulin G that recognizes the intracellular epitope of prostate-specific membrane antigen. Early (30 minutes after infusion) and delayed images (96–120 hours later) are taken with planar and cross-sectional single-photon emission tomography to identify areas of activity.

Since its approval by the US Food and Drug Administration, controversy has surrounded its appropriate use. Two important issues have not been fully resolved regarding the utility of indium 111 capromab pendetide scans in the rising PSA disease state. The first is the lack of comparison data between labeled antibody imaging and conventional imaging. Seltzer and colleagues [75] found that abdominal and pelvic helical CT scan (and whole-body FDG-PET scan) had a higher detection rate than labeled antibody imaging in patients who had a PSA greater than 4.0 ng/mL. Moreover, six patients had their metastasis proven by biopsy, yet only one of these six had a positive indium 111 capromab study in that area.

The second issue is the ability of indium 111 capromab scans to predict outcomes in men who undergo salvage radiation therapy to the prostate bed. Again, the results are controversial. Two studies (in 32 and 13 men, respectively) found that men who had a negative indium 111 capromab scan outside the pelvis had a statistically higher likelihood of a durable PSA response at 35 and 17 months, respectively, than those who had an abnormal scan outside the pelvis [76–78]. In the larger of the two trials, the only variable associated with a durable response to salvage radiotherapy was having a negative radiolabeled antibody scan outside the pelvis. On the other hand, a retrospective study of 30 men at the University of Michigan found no relationship between indium 111 capromab scans and response to salvage radiation therapy [79]. A smaller study also found poor durable response rates to salvage radiation therapy despite only localized uptake after radiolabeled antibody scan [80].

In summary, the added value of indium 111 capromab scans to conventional imaging and patient characteristics (Gleason score, serum PSA, time since surgery) in patients who have a rising PSA after radical prostatectomy has still not been con-clusively demonstrated. A randomized trial is needed, perhaps using coregistration of the radiola-beled antibody scan with abdominal/pelvic CT scans.

Bone scintigraphy

Unlike in clinically localized disease, much less data are available to guide the use of BS in the rising PSA setting. The following, however, are some guiding principles:

1. BS, as a method of following patients for pros-tate cancer recurrence before PSA elevation, is useless [81,82].
2. Patients who have a rising PSA and new, repro-ducible pain should undergo BS as an initial di-agnostic procedure regardless of the absolute PSA level [83].
3. Pain alone has poor sensitivity for predicting bone metastases [84]; therefore, in patients who have a rising PSA and are entering a trial that requires the absence of radiographic evi-dence of disease, BS should be done to ensure eligibility.

For asymptomatic men who have a rising PSA, the timing and frequency of BS is controversial. Sev-eral studies have considered this issue [85–87]. Some of the most informative data comes from Cher and colleagues [85]. They retrospectively re-viewed bone scans from 93 patients (most of whom were androgen sensitive) who had a rising PSA after radical prostatectomy. In a multivariate analysis, they found that serum PSA was the stron-gest predictor of a true positive BS. In men who had a PSA less than 40 ng/mL, the probability of a posi-tive BS was less than 5%. Other studies have found that a high PSA velocity (>0.5 ng/mL/mo) and an involved lymph node at radical prostatectomy are also predictors of a true positive BS [86]. A reason-able strategy in symptomatic, hormone-sensitive men who have a rising PSA is to use BS for screening only when the PSA has exceeded 30 to 40 ng/mL or when the PSA velocity is greater than 0.5 ng/mL/mo. This strategy should be used with caution, however, because these studies are small and the confidence intervals around the point estimate of BS positivity are large.

This strategy does not apply to men who have a rising PSA after androgen ablation. The data re-garding the appropriate timing of BS in this group are limited. Smith and colleagues [66] considered a cohort of 201 patients who had a rising PSA after androgen ablation but no evidence of metastatic disease on conventional imaging and followed them with BS every 4 months. After 2 years, only 33% had developed at least one bone metastasis. The predictors of time to first bone metastasis, which remained significant in a multivariate analy-sis, were baseline PSA greater than 10 ng/mL and a higher PSA velocity. In men who had a PSA less than 7.7 ng/mL at baseline or a PSA doubling time greater than 18.8 months, approximately 10% developed positive BS at 1 year. Thus, for men who have long PSA doubling times or low baseline serum PSA levels, a prolonged time be-tween BS screenings may be appropriate.

Use of 2-deoxy-2-[^{18}F]fluoro-D-glucose positron emission tomography

The use of FDG is limited by normal urinary excre-tion, resulting in high radioactivity within the blad-der and, therefore, image artifacts in the pelvis. This artifact may explain, in part, the initial negative studies in this disease state [88]. The use of furose-mide, continuous bladder irrigation, and newer it-erative image reconstruction has significantly improved this situation [89]. Two recent studies in particular have considered the role of FDG-PET with one of these methods in the biochemical re-lapse setting [75,90]. Overall, even with the use of bladder irrigation or newer iterative image recon-struction, it is unclear how much FDG-PET adds to conventional imaging (BS, erMR imaging) in pa-tients who have biochemically recurred after radical prostatectomy but are still good candidates for sal-vage radiotherapy (PSA <4.0 ng/mL). Perhaps the most interesting situation is when FDG-PET is neg-ative or negative outside the prostate bed: here it would be valuable to know whether a negative non-local FDG-PET predicts the success of salvage radio-therapy. Larger studies with long-term outcomes are needed to further define the role of FDG-PET in this setting.

Recommendations

The data for the use of any imaging tests in patients who have biochemical recurrence but no symptoms attributable to prostate cancer are very limited. In patients for whom the diagnosis of local recurrence will have an impact on treatment decisions, erMR imaging is a reasonable choice (especially after rad-ical prostatectomy). BS is needed only in the setting of symptoms, high PSA velocity, or an absolute PSA level greater than 30 to 40 ng/mL. More data are needed to properly define the role of radiolabeled antibody studies or PET.

Summary

Appropriate imaging for prostate cancer patients depends on the clinical disease state of the patient and the question being asked (Table 3). For

Table 3: Imaging recommendations

Disease state	Questions asked	Imaging modality
No cancer diagnosis	Does this patient have prostate cancer?	TRUS
Clinically localized disease	Does this patient have T3 disease? Does this patient have lymph node involvement? Does this patient have distant metastases?	BS and erMR imaging in patients with higher-risk disease
Rising PSA	Does this patient have local recurrence? Does this patient have distant metastases?	erMR imaging in patients who might benefit from local therapy; BS in patients who have higher PSA or PSA velocity

patients who do not have a cancer diagnosis, US is the standard approach, in combination with a sextant biopsy. In the future, contrast-enhanced US and MR imaging–directed biopsy may improve biopsy yield and decrease biopsy number. For patients who have clinically localized disease, erMR imaging and BS may play a role in patients who have risk factors for extracapsular extension, but more data are needed to define the role of MR spectroscopy and LNMR imaging. In the rising PSA setting, erMR imaging may help define local recurrence, whereas BS can be useful in the setting of a higher PSA or PSA velocity.

Important issues that remain for all trials of imaging modalities in prostate cancer include standardizing patient populations within trials, demonstrating the reproducibility of these techniques between different centers, and understanding how information gained should influence patient care. We eagerly await the answers to these questions.

References

[1] Jemal A, Murray T, Ward E, et al. Cancer statistics, 2005. CA Cancer J Clin 2005;55(1):10–30.

[2] Scher HI, Heller G. Clinical states in prostate cancer: toward a dynamic model of disease progression. Urology 2000;55(3):323–7.

[3] Scher HI, Eisenberger M, D'Amico AV, et al. Eligibility and outcomes reporting guidelines for clinical trials for patients in the state of a rising prostate-specific antigen: recommendations from the Prostate-Specific Antigen Working Group. J Clin Oncol 2004;22(3):537–56.

[4] Cooperberg MR, Lubeck DP, Meng MV, et al. The changing face of low-risk prostate cancer: trends in clinical presentation and primary management. J Clin Oncol 2004;22(11):2141–9.

[5] Coffield KS, Speights VO, Brawn PN, et al. Ultrasound detection of prostate cancer in postmortem specimens with histological correlation. J Urol 1992;147(3 Pt 2):822–6.

[6] Kuligowska E, Barish MA, Fenlon HM, et al. Predictors of prostate carcinoma: accuracy of gray-scale and color Doppler US and serum markers. Radiology 2001;220(3):757–64.

[7] Naughton CK, Miller DC, Mager DE, et al. A prospective randomized trial comparing 6 versus 12 prostate biopsy cores: impact on cancer detection. J Urol 2000;164(2):388–92.

[8] Stewart CS, Leibovich BC, Weaver AL, et al. Prostate cancer diagnosis using a saturation needle biopsy technique after previous negative sextant biopsies. J Urol 2001;166(1):86–91 [discussion: 91–82].

[9] Yu KK, Hricak H. Imaging prostate cancer. Radiol Clin North Am 2000;38(1):59–85 [viii].

[10] Purohit RS, Shinohara K, Meng MV, et al. Imaging clinically localized prostate cancer. Urol Clin North Am 2003;30(2):279–93.

[11] Leventis AK, Shariat SF, Utsunomiya T, et al. Characteristics of normal prostate vascular anatomy as displayed by power Doppler. Prostate 2001;46(4):281–8.

[12] Frauscher F, Klauser A, Halpern EJ, et al. Detection of prostate cancer with a microbubble ultrasound contrast agent. Lancet 2001;357(9271): 1849–50.

[13] Blomley M, Cosgrove D. Microbubble echo-enhancers: a new direction for ultrasound? Lancet 1997;349(9069):1855–6.

[14] Frauscher F, Halpern EJ, Klauser A. Accuracy of gray-scale and color Doppler US and serum markers as predictors of prostate carcinoma. Radiology 2002;223(1):282–3 [author reply: 283–4].

[15] Frauscher F, Klauser A, Volgger H, et al. Comparison of contrast enhanced color Doppler targeted biopsy with conventional systematic biopsy: impact on prostate cancer detection. J Urol 2002;167(4):1648–52.

[16] Albertsen PC, Hanley JA, Fine J. 20-year outcomes following conservative management of clinically localized prostate cancer. JAMA 2005; 293(17):2095–101.

[17] Prando A, Kurhanewicz J, Borges AP, et al. Prostatic biopsy directed with endorectal MR spectroscopic imaging findings in patients with elevated prostate specific antigen levels and prior negative biopsy findings: early experience. Radiology 2005;236(3):903–10.

[18] Messing EM, Manola J, Sarosdy M, et al. Immediate hormonal therapy compared with observation after radical prostatectomy and pelvic lymphadenectomy in men with node-positive prostate cancer. N Engl J Med 1999;341(24): 1781–8.

[19] Smith JA Jr, Scardino PT, Resnick MI, et al. Transrectal ultrasound versus digital rectal examination for the staging of carcinoma of the prostate: results of a prospective, multi-institutional trial. J Urol 1997;157(3):902–6.

[20] Engeler CE, Wasserman NF, Zhang G. Preoperative assessment of prostatic carcinoma by computerized tomography. Weaknesses and new perspectives. Urology 1992;40(4):346–50.

[21] Rifkin MD, Zerhouni EA, Gatsonis CA, et al. Comparison of magnetic resonance imaging and ultrasonography in staging early prostate cancer. Results of a multi-institutional cooperative trial. N Engl J Med 1990;323(10):621–6.

[22] Abuzallouf S, Dayes I, Lukka H. Baseline staging of newly diagnosed prostate cancer: a summary of the literature. J Urol 2004;171(6 Pt 1): 2122–7.

[23] Manyak MJ, Javitt MC. The role of computerized tomography, magnetic resonance imaging, bone scan, and monoclonal antibody nuclear scan for prognosis prediction in prostate cancer. Semin Urol Oncol 1998;16(3):145–52.

[24] Engelbrecht MR, Jager GJ, Laheij RJ, et al. Local staging of prostate cancer using magnetic resonance imaging: a meta-analysis. Eur Radiol 2002;12(9):2294–302.

[25] Tempany CM, Zhou X, Zerhouni EA, et al. Staging of prostate cancer: results of Radiology Diagnostic Oncology Group project comparison of three MR imaging techniques. Radiology 1994; 192(1):47–54.

[26] Bernstein MR, Cangiano T, D'Amico A, et al. Endorectal coil magnetic resonance imaging and clinicopathologic findings in T1c adenocarcinoma of the prostate. Urol Oncol 2000;5(3): 104–7.

[27] D'Amico AV, Whittington R, Malkowicz SB, et al. Critical analysis of the ability of the endorectal coil magnetic resonance imaging scan to predict pathologic stage, margin status, and postoperative prostate-specific antigen failure in patients with clinically organ-confined prostate cancer. J Clin Oncol 1996;14(6):1770–7.

[28] Cheng GC, Chen MH, Whittington R, et al. Clinical utility of endorectal MRI in determining PSA outcome for patients with biopsy Gleason score 7, PSA < or = 10, and clinically localized prostate cancer. Int J Radiat Oncol Biol Phys 2003; 55(1):64–70.

[29] D'Amico AV, Whittington R, Malkowicz B, et al. Endorectal magnetic resonance imaging as a predictor of biochemical outcome after radical prostatectomy in men with clinically localized prostate cancer. J Urol 2000;164(3 Pt 1):759–63.

[30] D'Amico AV, Whittington R, Malkowicz SB, et al. Combination of the preoperative PSA level, biopsy Gleason score, percentage of positive biopsies, and MRI T-stage to predict early PSA failure in men with clinically localized prostate cancer. Urology 2000;55(4):572–7.

[31] Brown G, Macvicar DA, Ayton V, et al. The role of intravenous contrast enhancement in magnetic resonance imaging of prostatic carcinoma. Clin Radiol 1995;50(9):601–6.

[32] Engelbrecht MR, Huisman HJ, Laheij RJ, et al. Discrimination of prostate cancer from normal peripheral zone and central gland tissue by using dynamic contrast-enhanced MR imaging. Radiology 2003;229(1):248–54.

[33] Hara N, Okuizumi M, Koike H, et al. Dynamic contrast-enhanced magnetic resonance imaging (DCE-MRI) is a useful modality for the precise detection and staging of early prostate cancer. Prostate 2005;62(2):140–7.

[34] Ito H, Kamoi K, Yokoyama K, et al. Visualization of prostate cancer using dynamic contrast-enhanced MRI: comparison with transrectal power Doppler ultrasound. Br J Radiol 2003; 76(909):617–24.

[35] Jager GJ, Ruijter ET, van de Kaa CA, et al. Dynamic TurboFLASH subtraction technique for contrast-enhanced MR imaging of the prostate: correlation with histopathologic results. Radiology 1997;203(3):645–52.

[36] Namimoto T, Morishita S, Saitoh R, et al. The value of dynamic MR imaging for hypointensity lesions of the peripheral zone of the prostate. Comput Med Imaging Graph 1998;22(3): 239–45.

[37] Ogura K, Maekawa S, Okubo K, et al. Dynamic endorectal magnetic resonance imaging for local staging and detection of neurovascular bundle involvement of prostate cancer: correlation with histopathologic results. Urology 2001;57(4): 721–6.

[38] Padhani AR, Gapinski CJ, Macvicar DA, et al. Dynamic contrast enhanced MRI of prostate cancer: correlation with morphology and tumour stage, histological grade and PSA. Clin Radiol 2000; 55(2):99–109.

[39] Coakley FV, Qayyum A, Kurhanewicz J. Magnetic resonance imaging and spectroscopic imaging of prostate cancer. J Urol 2003;170(6 Pt 2):S69–75 [discussion: S75–66].

[40] Kurhanewicz J, Vigneron DB, Hricak H, et al. Three-dimensional H-1 MR spectroscopic imaging of the in situ human prostate with high (0.24–0.7-cm3) spatial resolution. Radiology 1996;198(3):795–805.

[41] Kurhanewicz J, Vigneron DB, Nelson SJ. Three-dimensional magnetic resonance spectroscopic

imaging of brain and prostate cancer. Neoplasia 2000;2(1–2):166–89.

[42] Scheidler J, Hricak H, Vigneron DB, et al. Prostate cancer: localization with three-dimensional proton MR spectroscopic imaging—clinicopathologic study. Radiology 1999;213(2):473–80.

[43] Wefer AE, Hricak H, Vigneron DB, et al. Sextant localization of prostate cancer: comparison of sextant biopsy, magnetic resonance imaging and magnetic resonance spectroscopic imaging with step section histology. J Urol 2000;164(2): 400–4.

[44] Coakley FV, Kurhanewicz J, Lu Y, et al. Prostate cancer tumor volume: measurement with endorectal MR and MR spectroscopic imaging. Radiology 2002;223(1):91–7.

[45] Yu KK, Scheidler J, Hricak H, et al. Prostate cancer: prediction of extracapsular extension with endorectal MR imaging and three-dimensional proton MR spectroscopic imaging. Radiology 1999;213(2):481–8.

[46] Futterer JJ, Heijmink SW, Scheenen TW, et al. Prostate cancer: local staging at 3-T endorectal MR imaging—early experience. Radiology 2006; 238(1):184–91.

[47] Harisinghani MG, Saini S, Weissleder R, et al. MR lymphangiography using ultrasmall superparamagnetic iron oxide in patients with primary abdominal and pelvic malignancies: radiographic-pathologic correlation. AJR Am J Roentgenol 1999;172(5):1347–51.

[48] Weissleder R, Elizondo G, Wittenberg J, et al. Ultrasmall superparamagnetic iron oxide: an intravenous contrast agent for assessing lymph nodes with MR imaging. Radiology 1990;175(2): 494–8.

[49] Weissleder R, Elizondo G, Wittenberg J, et al. Ultrasmall superparamagnetic iron oxide: characterization of a new class of contrast agents for MR imaging. Radiology 1990;175(2):489–93.

[50] Harisinghani MG, Barentsz J, Hahn PF, et al. Noninvasive detection of clinically occult lymph-node metastases in prostate cancer. N Engl J Med 2003;348(25):2491–9.

[51] Hamaoka T, Madewell JE, Podoloff DA, et al. Bone imaging in metastatic breast cancer. J Clin Oncol 2004;22(14):2942–53.

[52] Even-Sapir E. Imaging of malignant bone involvement by morphologic, scintigraphic, and hybrid modalities. J Nucl Med 2005;46(8): 1356–67.

[53] Shvarts O, Han KR, Seltzer M, et al. Positron emission tomography in urologic oncology. Cancer Control 2002;9(4):335–42.

[54] Kumar R, Zhuang H, Alavi A. PET in the management of urologic malignancies. Radiol Clin North Am 2004;42(6):1141–53 [ix].

[55] Schoder H, Larson SM. Positron emission tomography for prostate, bladder, and renal cancer. Semin Nucl Med 2004;34(4):274–92.

[56] de Jong IJ, Pruim J, Elsinga PH, et al. Preoperative staging of pelvic lymph nodes in prostate cancer by 11C-choline PET. J Nucl Med 2003; 44(3):331–5.

[57] Oyama N, Akino H, Kanamaru H, et al. 11C-acetate PET imaging of prostate cancer. J Nucl Med 2002;43(2):181–6.

[58] Liu IJ, Zafar MB, Lai YH, et al. Fluorodeoxyglucose positron emission tomography studies in diagnosis and staging of clinically organ-confined prostate cancer. Urology 2001;57(1): 108–11.

[59] Effert PJ, Bares R, Handt S, et al. Metabolic imaging of untreated prostate cancer by positron emission tomography with 18fluorine-labeled deoxyglucose. J Urol 1996;155(3):994–8.

[60] Sanz G, Robles JE, Gimenez M, et al. Positron emission tomography with 18fluorine-labelled deoxyglucose: utility in localized and advanced prostate cancer. BJU Int 1999;84(9):1028–31.

[61] Oyama N, Akino H, Suzuki Y, et al. The increased accumulation of [18F]fluorodeoxyglucose in untreated prostate cancer. Jpn J Clin Oncol 1999; 29(12):623–9.

[62] Heicappell R, Muller-Mattheis V, Reinhardt M, et al. Staging of pelvic lymph nodes in neoplasms of the bladder and prostate by positron emission tomography with 2-[(18)F]-2-deoxy-D-glucose. Eur Urol 1999;36(6):582–7.

[63] Kato T, Tsukamoto E, Kuge Y, et al. Accumulation of [11C]acetate in normal prostate and benign prostatic hyperplasia: comparison with prostate cancer. Eur J Nucl Med Mol Imaging 2002; 29(11):1492–5.

[64] Kotzerke J, Volkmer BG, Glatting G, et al. Intra-individual comparison of [11C]acetate and [11C]choline PET for detection of metastases of prostate cancer. Nuklearmedizin 2003;42(1): 25–30.

[65] Pound CR, Partin AW, Eisenberger MA, et al. Natural history of progression after PSA elevation following radical prostatectomy. JAMA 1999;281(17):1591–7.

[66] Smith MR, Kabbinavar F, Saad F, et al. Natural history of rising serum prostate-specific antigen in men with castrate nonmetastatic prostate cancer. J Clin Oncol 2005;23(13):2918–25.

[67] Stephenson AJ, Shariat SF, Zelefsky MJ, et al. Salvage radiotherapy for recurrent prostate cancer after radical prostatectomy. JAMA 2004;291(11): 1325–32.

[68] Hricak H, Schoder H, Pucar D, et al. Advances in imaging in the postoperative patient with a rising prostate-specific antigen level. Semin Oncol 2003;30(5):616–34.

[69] Sella T, Schwartz LH, Swindle PW, et al. Suspected local recurrence after radical prostatectomy: endorectal coil MR imaging. Radiology 2004;231(2):379–85.

[70] Silverman JM, Krebs TL. MR imaging evaluation with a transrectal surface coil of local recurrence of prostatic cancer in men who have undergone radical prostatectomy. AJR Am J Roentgenol 1997;168(2):379–85.

[71] Chan TW, Kressel HY. Prostate and seminal vesicles after irradiation: MR appearance. J Magn Reson Imaging 1991;1(5):503–11.

[72] Coakley FV, Hricak H, Wefer AE, et al. Brachytherapy for prostate cancer: endorectal MR imaging of local treatment-related changes. Radiology 2001;219(3):817–21.

[73] Sala E, Eberhardt SC, Akin O, et al. Endorectal MR imaging before salvage prostatectomy: tumor localization and staging. Radiology 2006; 238(1):176–83.

[74] Coakley FV, Teh HS, Qayyum A, et al. Endorectal MR imaging and MR spectroscopic imaging for locally recurrent prostate cancer after external beam radiation therapy: preliminary experience. Radiology 2004;233(2):441–8.

[75] Seltzer MA, Barbaric Z, Belldegrun A, et al. Comparison of helical computerized tomography, positron emission tomography and monoclonal antibody scans for evaluation of lymph node metastases in patients with prostate specific antigen relapse after treatment for localized prostate cancer. J Urol 1999;162(4):1322–8.

[76] Kahn D, Williams RD, Haseman MK, et al. Radioimmunoscintigraphy with In-111-labeled capromab pendetide predicts prostate cancer response to salvage radiotherapy after failed radical prostatectomy. J Clin Oncol 1998;16(1): 284–9.

[77] Levesque PE, Nieh PT, Zinman LN, et al. Radiolabeled monoclonal antibody indium 111-labeled CYT-356 localizes extraprostatic recurrent carcinoma after prostatectomy. Urology 1998;51(6): 978–84.

[78] Kahn D, Austin J, Miller S, et al. IN-111 capromab pendetide MAB scan predicts response to radiotherapy to the prostate fossa in men with tumor recurrence following radical prostatectomy: 3-years follow-up. J Urol 1999;161(4S): 239.

[79] Thomas CT, Bradshaw PT, Pollock BH, et al. Indium-111-capromab pendetide radioimmunoscintigraphy and prognosis for durable biochemical response to salvage radiation therapy in men after failed prostatectomy. J Clin Oncol 2003;21(9):1715–21.

[80] Wilkinson S, Chodak G. The role of 111indium-capromab pendetide imaging for assessing biochemical failure after radical prostatectomy. J Urol 2004;172(1):133–6.

[81] Terris MK, Klonecke AS, McDougall IR, et al. Utilization of bone scans in conjunction with prostate-specific antigen levels in the surveillance for recurrence of adenocarcinoma after radical prostatectomy. J Nucl Med 1991;32(9):1713–7.

[82] Miller PD, Eardley I, Kirby RS. Prostate specific antigen and bone scan correlation in the staging and monitoring of patients with prostatic cancer. Br J Urol 1992;70(3):295–8.

[83] Lee CT, Oesterling JE. Using prostate-specific antigen to eliminate the staging radionuclide bone scan. Urol Clin North Am 1997;24(2):389–94.

[84] Palmer E, Henrikson B, McKusick K, et al. Pain as an indicator of bone metastasis. Acta Radiol 1988;29(4):445–9.

[85] Cher ML, Bianco FJ Jr, Lam JS, et al. Limited role of radionuclide bone scintigraphy in patients with prostate specific antigen elevations after radical prostatectomy. J Urol 1998;160(4):1387–91.

[86] Kane CJ, Amling CL, Johnstone PA, et al. Limited value of bone scintigraphy and computed tomography in assessing biochemical failure after radical prostatectomy. Urology 2003;61(3): 607–11.

[87] Partin AW, Pearson JD, Landis PK, et al. Evaluation of serum prostate-specific antigen velocity after radical prostatectomy to distinguish local recurrence from distant metastases. Urology 1994;43(5):649–59.

[88] Hofer C, Laubenbacher C, Block T, et al. Fluorine-18-fluorodeoxyglucose positron emission tomography is useless for the detection of local recurrence after radical prostatectomy. Eur Urol 1999;36(1):31–5.

[89] Turlakow A, Larson SM, Coakley F, et al. Local detection of prostate cancer by positron emission tomography with 2-fluorodeoxyglucose: comparison of filtered back projection and iterative reconstruction with segmented attenuation correction. Q J Nucl Med 2001;45(3):235–44.

[90] Schoder H, Herrmann K, Gonen M, et al. 2-[18F]fluoro-2-deoxyglucose positron emission tomography for the detection of disease in patients with prostate-specific antigen relapse after radical prostatectomy. Clin Cancer Res 2005; 11(13):4761–9.

ELSEVIER
SAUNDERS

RADIOLOGIC
CLINICS
OF NORTH AMERICA

Radiol Clin N Am 44 (2006) 723–734

MR Imaging and MR Spectroscopy in Prostate Cancer Management

Sharyn Katz, MD, Mark Rosen, MD, PhD*

- Role of MR imaging in prostate cancer diagnosis
- Endorectal coil MR imaging techniques and cancer detection
- MR imaging for depiction of known prostate cancer
- Staging of prostate cancer
- MR imaging for local staging of prostate cancer
- MR spectroscopy and MR spectroscopic imaging
  Added value for MR spectroscopic imaging for local tumor staging
- Future improvement in MR imaging: 3 T, new coils

- Current trends in management of localized prostate cancer
  MR imaging/MR spectroscopic imaging and radiation therapy planning
- Cancer localization
  MR imaging-guided biopsy
- Newer MR imaging techniques
  Dynamic contrast-enhanced MR imaging
  Diffusion-weighted imaging
- Multimodality MR imaging of prostate cancer
- Nodal staging: routine plus ultrasmall superparamagnetic iron oxide
- Post therapy/recurrence
- Summary
- References

Prostate cancer continues to be a major health concern in the United States. In 2005, there were 232,090 new cases of prostate cancer and 30,350 deaths secondary to prostate cancer [1]. Prostate cancer continues to be diagnosed with increasing frequency [2], although overall, there has been a slight decline in mortality in the past decade [3]. With the advent of screening by way of prostate-specific antigen (PSA), most prostate cancers are detected at an early stage [4]. Early detection, however, may not always translate into improved outcomes. The biologic activity of prostate cancer is variable, and the time course between the appearance of detectable tumor and disseminated disease spread can vary widely. Furthermore, autopsy series demonstrate that many men who die from other causes are found to have indolent prostate cancer. It is therefore understood that some men who receive the diagnosis of prostate cancer harbor disease that left untreated, would not negatively affect mortality or cause morbidity [5]. Consequently, there is much interest in identifying markers of disease activity that would predict which localized cancers are destined to be more biologically aggressive.

Role of MR imaging in prostate cancer diagnosis

The role of MR imaging in the diagnosis, staging, and follow-up of prostate cancer remains widely debated in the urologic community. The advent of the endorectal coil [6] for high-resolution imaging of

Department of Radiology, University of Pennsylvania Medical Center, 3400 Spruce Street, Philadelphia, PA 19104
* Corresponding author.
E-mail address: rosenmar@uphs.upenn.edu (M. Rosen).

0033-8389/06/$ – see front matter © 2006 Elsevier Inc. All rights reserved.
radiologic.theclinics.com

doi:10.1016/j.rcl.2006.07.008

the prostate was hailed as a major achievement in prostate cancer imaging, but even with endorectal coil imaging, many small tumors may not be readily detectable by MR imaging; thus, few investigators advocate the use of MR imaging as a screening tool for prostate cancer. In patients who have elevated PSA and negative biopsy, however, MR imaging with endorectal coil has been shown to be useful in predicting which patients are likely to have cancer detected on a subsequent biopsy [7,8]. Nevertheless, in centers at which endorectal coil MR imaging of the prostate is used, it is almost exclusively used as a staging tool for men who have recently diagnosed cancer. The overall use of MR imaging in the evaluation of newly diagnosed prostate cancer varies nationally [9].

Endorectal coil MR imaging techniques and cancer detection

With endorectal coil MR imaging, the detector coil is placed immediately adjacent to the prostate gland (Fig. 1). This geometry optimizes signal from the posterior and posterolateral aspects of the prostate gland. For larger prostate glands, the rapid fall-off of the receptive profile of the local endorectal coil is compensated for by the inclusion of anterior external-array pelvic coils so that a more uniform image of the prostate is obtained. Automated intensity correction schemes can further improve the homogeneity of the image [10].

In prostate MR imaging, high-resolution T2-weighted (T2W) imaging is used to identify tumor in the prostate and the spread of tumor into the adjacent periprostatic tissues. The normal peripheral zone (PZ) of the prostate is bright on T2W images

(Fig. 2). Tumor in the PZ is darker on these same images, allowing for depiction of cancer at high resolution (Fig. 3). Several factors complicate the evaluation of the prostate on T2W imaging. With aging, noncancerous changes in the PZ (such as scarring from prostatitis) alter the normal bright background of the PZ. Aging also leads to variable degrees of benign prostatic hypertrophy (BPH), causing central gland enlargement. In more severe cases of BPH, the PZ can be severely compressed by the enlarging central gland compromising depiction of cancer in the PZ (Fig. 4). Changes associated with BPH in the central gland can be variable, depending on the balance between stromal and glandular elements of prostatic hypertrophy (Fig. 5). This variegated appearance of BPH on T2 imaging makes detection of central gland tumor (which can occur in roughly 25% of cases) more difficult.

MR imaging for depiction of known prostate cancer

Most prostate cancers are identified clinically by transrectal ultrasound (TRUS)-guided biopsy, usually performed for an elevated screening PSA or an abnormal finding on digital rectal examination in the absence of PSA elevation. MR imaging is usually performed for staging after the diagnosis of prostate cancer has been established. Postbiopsy hemorrhage within the prostate gland is therefore often seen on the MR imaging, further complicating the task of tumor depiction on MR imaging because hemorrhage can also lead to T2W signal abnormality in the PZ of the prostate gland [11]. However, hemorrhage can easily be identified through the use of supplemental T1-weighted (T1W) imaging.

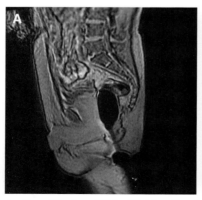 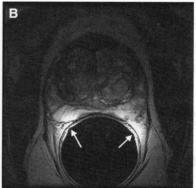

Fig. 1. Endorectal coil positioning. (*A*) Sagittal localizer image demonstrates correct placement of the endorectal coil. The coil is placed within the rectum and advanced toward the prostate. The balloon is then expanded to fill the rectum, which immobilizes the coil and places the coil detector elements immediately against the posterior aspect of the prostate gland. (*B*) Axial T2-weighted image demonstrates the appearance of the rectum with the coil balloon expanded. The coil elements are the bright areas or "hot-spots"(*arrows*) at the lateral aspects of the anterior rectal wall.

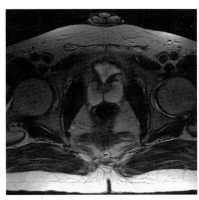

Fig. 2. Normal prostate. Axial T2W pelvic image from a 22-year-old man undergoing MR evaluation for scrotal abnormality. The normal appearance of the prostate, with a bright uniform PZ, is demonstrated.

Paired T2W and T1W images of the prostate can be coinspected (Fig. 6). A T2W signal abnormality shown to be secondary to hemorrhage on T1W images is not deemed suspicious for tumor. Because hemorrhage does not extend into the tumor nodules, the nodules are often outlined by the blood (the so-called "hemorrhage exclusion sign") (Fig. 7).

In most men who undergo prostate MR imaging for staging of known cancer, there is coexisting benign disease (BPH, prostatitis). These findings can alter the homogeneity of noncancerous PZ tissue on T2W imaging, complicating the depiction of smaller tumor nodules. Even larger tumors may be difficult to identify. In one study, only approximately 70% of tumor nodules greater than 0.5 cm^3 were correctly identified on endorectal prostate

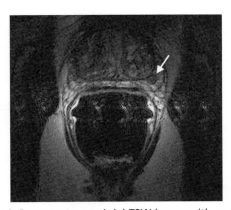

Fig. 3. Prostate cancer. Axial T2W image with endorectal coil demonstrates a small round focus of dark signal in the left PZ (*arrow*). Transrectal ultrasound–guided biopsy revealed left-sided carcinoma. Subsequent prostatectomy revealed a single cancer focus on the left, Gleason score 6, with no capsular extension or spread.

MR imaging [12]. The detection rate is likely lower for even smaller tumors. These findings suggest that prostate MR imaging is unlikely to serve as an adequate screening modality for prostate cancer. It remains to be determined, however, whether cancers that are occult on MR imaging are as clinically significant as those that are larger and, hence, more readily detected on MR imaging.

Staging of prostate cancer

Initial staging of prostate cancer is a key component toward determining the appropriate therapy. The staging system most widely used is the TNM system (Box 1). This staging system is based on the extent of cancer within the prostate, the presence or absence of disease beyond the prostate gland (including local organ invasion), and the presence or absence of nodal or distant metastatic disease.

Local staging of the tumor is the most germane issue for treatment planning. In particular, the presence or absence of extension of tumor beyond the prostate capsule is considered a key factor for choosing between surgical and nonsurgical therapy. Because surgical margin status has been shown to be an independent predictor of disease recurrence [13], patients who have only minimal extracapsular disease may still benefit from surgical therapy. In patients who have more advanced extracapsular disease, there is an increased likelihood of tumor relapse after surgery [14]. Assessing for the presence or absence of seminal vesicle invasion is of particular importance because it is a strong predictor of subsequent development of locally recurrent or distant metastatic disease [15].

To facilitate the prediction of organ-confined disease estimates for individual patients, a nomogram was developed [16]. The Partin nomogram requires three pieces of information: clinical stage (ie, digital rectal examination assessment), Gleason grade of biopsy specimen, and PSA. Using these factors, one can estimate the likelihood of organ-confined disease in an individual, aiding in the determination of optimal surgical or nonsurgical management.

MR imaging for local staging of prostate cancer

Given the importance of extracapsular disease as a prognostic factor, there have been extensive efforts at studying the utility of endorectal coil MR imaging in identifying patients who have organ-confined or non–organ-confined disease [17]. The ability of MR imaging to depict extracapsular spread of tumor into the periprostatic fat depends on the amount of extracapsular tumor. Visualizing the direct extension of tumor into the fat is the clearest sign of

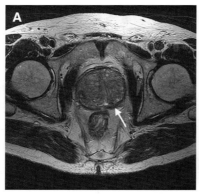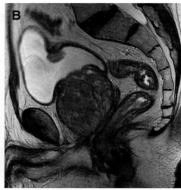

Fig. 4. BPH. Axial (*A*) and sagittal (*B*) T2W images demonstrate a markedly enlarged prostate gland. The PZ is seen as a nearly effaced linear band of tissue (*arrow in A*).

extracapsular disease on MR imaging. Secondary signs that are also associated with extracapsular disease include asymmetric capsular bulging, obliteration of the rectoprostatic angle, and involvement of the neurovascular bundle.

The ability of MR imaging to provide added clinical value beyond that offered by the Partin nomogram depends on the risk category of the patient [18,19]. In patients who have extremely low-risk for extracapsular disease (Gleason grade 2–4 and PSA <4.0 ng/mL), MR imaging probably has little added utility. In addition, in patients at extremely high risk for extracapsular disease (Gleason grade 8–10, PSA >20.0 ng/mL), the benefit of MR imaging remains uncertain. For those who have more moderate risk, however, MR imaging appears useful in

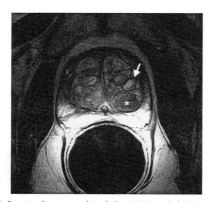

Fig. 5. Stromal versus glandular BPH. Axial T2W image with endorectal coil demonstrating the heterogeneous character of BPH. Image contrast is adjusted to highlight the texture of the central gland. Multinodular character of enlarged central gland is shown. Brighter nodules (*arrow*) correspond to glandular prostatic hypertrophy. Darker nodules (*asterisk*) denote areas of stromal dominant tissue. Appearance of stromal areas of BPH on T2W imaging overlaps with that of prostate carcinoma.

predicting true pathologic stage. In these cases, MR imaging can be used to identify those patients truly likely to benefit from surgery [20]. MR imaging can also aid in surgical planning for those who have marginal degrees of capsular penetration, such as aiding the urologist in defining whether nerve-sparing surgery would be an appropriate option [21].

MR spectroscopy and MR spectroscopic imaging

In MR spectroscopic imaging (MRSI), magnetic resonances signals of small molecular-weight metabolites that reside in tissues are revealed. These metabolites must be present in sufficient concentration (usually 1mM or greater) to be observable. Furthermore, the MR signal from bulk water (which is present at approximately 110 M, or roughly 10^5 times that of metabolites) must be suppressed, so that the weaker MR signals from these cellular metabolites may become visible.

The metabolites visualized in MRSI are identified by their resonance frequency, which is based on the chemical environment of the hydrogen atoms. Each metabolite resonates at a slightly different frequency, often referred to as chemical shift, which is measured in parts per million (ppm). MR spectroscopy is often used in the brain to detect characteristic metabolic signals (particularly *N*-acetyl aspartate) that are commonly found in neuronal tissue.

In prostate MR spectroscopy, several key metabolic resonances are identifiable. Principle among these is that of citrate, a metabolite found in relatively high concentrations in prostate tissue owing to its presence in prostatic secretions. The citrate resonance is found at 2.6 ppm. Other resonances of interest are creatine and choline, the latter being a metabolite that is often elevated in malignant tissue. These metabolites resonate at 3.0 and

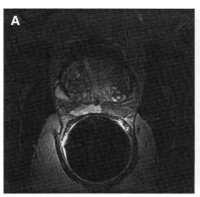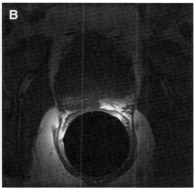

Fig. 6. Postbiopsy hemorrhage. (*A*) Axial T2W image with endorectal coil reveals varied bright and dark appearance within the PZ. Because both tumor and hemorrhage can be dark on T2W imaging, it is difficult to differentiate between postbiopsy change and tumor based solely on the T2W image. (*B*) Axial T1W image with endorectal coil. Image matrix, field of view, and slice location are identical to that of panel *A*. Coinspection of the T2W and T1W images reveals that all T2W dark areas of PZ demonstrate bright signal on the T1W image, confirming that the changes are related solely to postbiopsy hemorrhage.

3.2 ppm, respectively. Depending on the quality of the prostate MR spectroscopy examination, these resonance peaks may overlap partially. In addition, resonances from polyamines (another component of prostatic secretions) are also found in this region. As such, distinct choline and creatine resonances may merge and be hard to identify as separate peaks in the MR spectra.

In MRSI, the location of the spectrum or spectra in question is usually identified by a box or grid overlaid on an anatomic images (Fig. 8). MR spectroscopy can be performed as a single voxel over a specified lesion, or can be performed to obtain multiple spectra from a two-dimensional or three-dimensional grid. In prostate MRSI, a three-dimensional MRSI grid to encompass the entire prostate is usually performed.

MRSI of the prostate allows the reader to obtain metabolic information from distinct regions of the prostate gland. Because normal and cancerous prostate tissue contains distinct MR spectral signatures, the information from MRSI can be used to supplement that of MR imaging to identify areas of tumor involvement in the prostate. MRSI in conjunction with conventional MR imaging has been found to increase the number of cancers that can be detected [22,23] over that of standard MR imaging alone.

Added value for MR spectroscopic imaging for local tumor staging

Given the larger "voxel sizes" (in the range of 0.2–0.7 cm^3) of spectroscopic imaging, the resolution of prostate MRSI is not equivalent to that of MR imaging. Therefore, MRSI on its own cannot

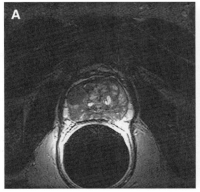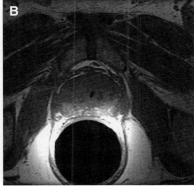

Fig. 7. Hemorrhage exclusion sign. (*A*) Axial T2W image with endorectal coil reveals multiple foci of dark signal in the PZ. On the T1W image at the same location (*B*), most of these areas are bright, representing postbiopsy hemorrhage; however, a single nodule in the anterior right PZ is seen that remains dark and appears to exclude the blood in the surrounding PZ on T1W imaging, suggesting tumor. TRUS-guided biopsy before imaging revealed right-sided tumor in several cores.

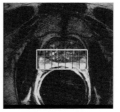

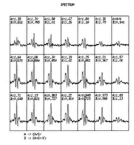

Fig. 8. MR spectroscopic imaging. Typical output of a prostate MRSI overlay. The axial T2W image is shown in the upper left. The MRSI grid is overlaid on the image. The outer white box is the user-defined boundary of the spatial-spectral saturation designed to limit lipid contamination from the periprostatic region. The inner boxes show the location of the MRSI voxels. On the right, the MRSI grid results show the spectra and calculated metabolite ratios.

smaller prostate cancers is less than optimal, and clear depiction of subtle degrees of extracapsular spread of tumor remains a challenge. If MR imaging is to become a more accepted modality for depiction and local staging of prostate cancer, then improvements in imaging accuracy are required. Two such advancements are the use of higher–field strength imaging (at 3 T) and improved coil design. The advantage of 3-T imaging lies chiefly in the gain in signal-to-noise relative to imaging at 1.5 T. Improvements in coil design include the use of rigid coils with higher signal and the introduction of a susceptibility-matched agent into the rectum to reduce distortions relating to the interface of rectal air and tissue.

The advantages of improved signal-to-noise secondary to coil improvements and 3-T imaging can be translated into higher-resolution imaging or faster scanning times. Faster scanning may help to reduce image artifacts related to patient motion and rectal peristalsis. Faster anatomic imaging also facilitates the incorporation of physiologic MR measures described later in this article, which may supplement anatomic imaging to depict prostate cancer more accurately.

Most critically, with improved signal-to-noise, higher-resolution imaging is possible [25,26]. It is expected that as imaging resolution improves, smaller tumors and more infiltrative tumors will become apparent, thus improving the performance of prostate MR imaging in cancer imaging.

depict small foci of extracapsular spread and cannot be used in isolation for staging of extracapsular spread of disease. Using MRSI as a supplement to conventional T2W MR imaging, however, can improve overall tumor depiction, which in turn may improve readers' confidence in identifying foci of extracapsular disease associated with smaller tumors that may have gone unrecognized on conventional T2W imaging alone. Thus, incorporation of MRSI with MR imaging may improve overall staging by distinguishing between organ-confined and extracapsular spread of disease [24].

Future improvement in MR imaging: 3 T, new coils

Endorectal coil prostate MR imaging has acknowledged limitations. Sensitivity for detection of

Current trends in management of localized prostate cancer

For prostate cancer that is confined to the prostate gland, there are various management options.

Surgical management through radical prostatectomy is often offered as a means to achieve cure. Radical prostatectomy, however, is generally not offered to patients whose life expectancy is gauged to be 10 years or less (ie, for patients who are likely to die of other causes before their prostate cancer would be expected to manifest clinically). Radical prostatectomy may also be contraindicated in patients who cannot tolerate major surgery (eg, severe cardiac or pulmonary compromise).

Radiation therapy is an alternative management option for patients who have confined disease for whom surgery is not indicated. Radiation therapy can be delivered externally or through brachytherapy implants of radioactive seeds. Traditionally, with external beam radiation therapy or brachytherapy, the therapeutic dose is distributed across the entire prostate gland, with a somewhat lower dose to the urethra. Care is taken to ensure that bystander organs (ie, rectum and bladder) receive lower does of therapy to avoid unwanted toxicity.

More recently, conservative management (so-called "watchful waiting") has been proposed as a viable alternative for patients who have early-stage lower-grade tumors. In watchful waiting, patients are carefully watched for signs of disease progression by way of serial PSA and follow-up biopsy.

MR imaging/MR spectroscopic imaging and radiation therapy planning

When radical prostatectomy is not indicated or when a patient prefers nonsurgical therapy, radiation therapy is often implemented. Whether the therapy is delivered internally by way of radioactive seed placement (brachytherapy) or externally, the goal of radiation therapy is to deliver a lethal dose of radiation to the tumor while sparing noncancerous tissues (especially those outside of the prostate) the cytotoxic doses of radiation that can lead to complications and increase patient morbidity.

Traditionally, radiation dose, whether internal by way of seed placement or external, is designed to encompass the entire prostate gland, with some dose sparing of the periurethral area. Radiation therapy planning therefore encompasses the creation of an anatomic map of the prostate and surrounding organs. This is generally done by way of CT. With the advent of MR imaging/MRSI for intraprostatic tumor localization, there has been a push to focus the higher doses of radiation to the tumor within the prostate, especially with the improvements in dose contouring of externally delivered radiation through intensity-modulated radiation therapy [27–29]. Improvements in intraprostatic tumor depiction by MR imaging/MRSI have aided this process [30,31]. The inflated balloon of the endorectal MR imaging coil, however, causes displacement and deformation of the prostate. Therefore, adequate treatment of tumor depicted by MR imaging (and avoidance of higher dose to susceptible bystander tissues such as rectal mucosa) requires the clinician to map the MR imaging/MRSI tumor locations correctly to the prostate in its "natural" state (ie, without rectal expansion). This is an active area of research in the radiation oncology field [32–34].

Of perhaps greater interest is the potential of real time MR imaging to guide brachytherapy seed placement [35–40]. The high resolution and tissue contrast of MR imaging can improve seed localization during the procedure, thus improving dose distribution to the tumor, the prostate as a whole, and the surrounding tissues. The high cost of MR imaging together with the technical impediments of implementing interventional MR imaging in the radiation oncology setting, however, have limited this application.

Cancer localization

MR imaging–guided biopsy

Currently, TRUS-guided biopsy is the mainstay for image-guided biopsy of the prostate in patients suspected to have prostate cancer. Ultrasound guidance is simple to use and relatively cost effective. By contrast, less attention has been paid to the use of MR imaging to guide biopsy. MR imaging guidance for biopsy, although technically feasible, remains a challenge, largely due to issues with patient access, patient positioning, and added cost. Nevertheless, MR imaging–guided biopsy procedures have been described [35,36,38]. The advantage of MR imaging guidance is the relatively improved depiction of cancer, thus facilitating accurate biopsy targeting and potentially decreasing the false-negative biopsy rate.

An alternative approach is the use of real-time software that allows the T2W MR image to be fused to the sonographic image during TRUS. In this scenario, the T2W MR image is overlaid on the sonographic image to target the area of tumor [35,41]. This technique may also improve the accuracy of TRUS and decrease the number of false-negative biopsy procedures, although the use of this technique has not been reported in any large series.

Newer MR imaging techniques

Dynamic contrast-enhanced MR imaging

In early reports of MR imaging for prostate cancer, it was shown that gadolinium-enhanced imaging was not helpful for detecting prostate cancer and was inferior to T2W imaging for delineating the location and extent of tumors [42]. These studies, however, evaluated only non–dynamic ("steady-state")-enhanced imaging, in which T1W imaging is performed before and 1 minute or several minutes after administration of intravenous gadolinium contrast agent. With the advent of faster MR scanning techniques, dynamic contrast-enhanced (DCE) MR imaging is increasingly being used for tissue and tumor characterization. DCE MR imaging uses rapid T1W imaging to monitor the signal intensity changes of tissue during the passage of contrast following rapid intravenous bolus administration. DCE MR imaging offers several potential advantages over steady-state imaging. Tumors, which enhance more rapidly than nonmalignant tissues, may be highlighted with better contrast during the early phase of DCE MR imaging, whereas imaging at later phases (such as is done in steady-state contrast-enhanced imaging) may demonstrate lower contrast between normal and malignant tissue. In addition, subtle differences between tumor and normal tissue, such as faster contrast wash-in or wash-out rates, may be highlighted through the generation of parametric "maps" from the series of DCE MR images.

Quantitative analysis of DCE MR imaging of prostate cancer has shown that cancers enhance more rapidly than noncancerous PZ tissue [43–45]. DCE MR imaging values of prostate cancer have also been reported to correlate with histologic assessment of neovascularity, such as tumor microvascular density [46]. Several reports have demonstrated the possible usefulness of DCE MR imaging in identifying areas of more rapid or intense tumor enhancement that are occult on routine T2W imaging [47]. DCE MR imaging has also been reported to aid in the staging of prostate cancer by highlighting areas of more rapid enhancement at sites of extracapsular disease [48]. DCE MR imaging is also an example of physiologic imaging. As such, quantification of DCE MR imaging parameters may allow for depiction of tumor biologic activity or prove useful in monitoring response to nonsurgical therapy.

Diffusion-weighted imaging

Diffusion-weighted MR imaging uses balanced positive and negative gradients to diphase and subsequently rephase water proton resonances before signal detection. When the motion of water molecules is heavily restricted, the gradient refocusing is optimized by the balanced gradients and no net signal loss due to dephasing occurs. If water freely diffuses along the direction of the gradient, then there is a net phase loss (or gain), which diminishes the signal within that portion of the tissue. By repeating the imaging at several different diffusion-gradient strengths, the apparent diffusion coefficient (ADC) at each voxel can be calculated. Diffusion-weighted imaging is commonly used to detect alteration in

water diffusion in areas of pathology, most notably in areas of cerebral ischemia during acute stroke.

Because the cellular structure of malignant tumors differs from that of normal tissue, it is expected that the diffusion of water will also differ in malignant versus nonmalignant tissues. Cancer growth may disrupt the glandular architecture, further altering water diffusion. Preliminary studies have addressed the feasibility of diffusion-weighted imaging for detecting prostate cancer. Several reports have shown that the ADC of prostate cancers is lower than that of unaffected PZ tissue [49–51]. It remains to be seen, however, whether the ADC maps themselves add value beyond routine T2 imaging in detecting prostate cancer. Additional studies are also required to evaluate whether ADC maps prove useful in detecting central gland tumor. It also remains to be seen whether the physiologic information from diffusion-weighted imaging correlates with the grade of prostate cancer and whether diffusion-weighted imaging may play a role in monitoring short- and long-term response to nonsurgical therapies.

Multimodality MR imaging of prostate cancer

With the advent of newer MR modalities such as spectroscopy, diffusion, and DCE MR imaging, the concept of "multimodal" MR imaging has arisen [52]. In this scheme, morphologic assessment through T2W imaging serves as a starting point rather than an end point for tumor detection. Multiple "physiologic" or "functional" layers can be added to the morphologic scaffolding of T2W images, with information derived from spectroscopy, DCE MR imaging, and diffusion. In theory, these added layers of information would improve the sensitivity and specificity of MR imaging for prostate cancer depiction and staging by providing the radiologist with additional information beyond that of T2W image intensity and image texture.

With the number of emerging techniques in MR imaging, the opportunity for computer-assisted detection (CAD) of prostate cancer by MR imaging is also growing. CAD has been studied as a means to augment the accuracy of radiologists' interpretation of screening mammograms, and several commercialized versions of CAD for mammography have been introduced. Given the wealth of information in prostate MR imaging examinations (morphologic and functional), CAD algorithms have been reported to improve the ability of radiologists to identify tumor compared with those of "single modality." These efforts remain preliminary, and most reports are limited to small pilot studies at single institutions. Additional research, however, may help define future MR imaging applications in disease staging and monitoring of nonsurgical therapy.

Nodal staging: routine plus ultrasmall superparamagnetic iron oxide

An additional area of prostate cancer staging not often addressed specifically by MR imaging is that of regional nodal staging. Although many cancers present at early stages when disease is expected to be organ confined or locally advanced into the periprostatic tissues, the possibility of nodal metastases must be considered in all higher- and intermediate-risk patients. The presence of nodal disease indicates a stage of cancer for which surgical therapy is not likely to benefit the patient.

It is unfortunate that the accuracy of routine cross-sectional imaging (CT or MR imaging) for identifying nodal disease is poor. Although enlargement of lymph nodes at key anatomic sites (eg, iliac and obturator regions) is specific for nodal spread of tumor, the sensitivity of cross-sectional imaging for detecting nodal disease is relatively low. This low sensitivity arises from the fact that lymph nodes which appear normal in size and shape by standard cross-sectional imaging may still harbor small foci of metastatic carcinoma. Retroperitoneal lymph node dissection with perioperative frozen tissue analysis, as is commonly performed as a precursor to radical prostatectomy, often depicts metastatic involvement in otherwise normal-appearing lymph nodes.

More recently, a newer class of MR contrast agents, the ultrasmall superparamagnetic iron oxide (USPIO) particles, has been developed. These small iron oxide particles are sequestered by lymph nodes and other tissues of the reticuloendothelial system as they circulate following intravenous administration. The effects of the iron oxide can be seen as signal loss on susceptibility (T2*) weighted gradient echo imaging. Thus, the reticuloendothelial functionality of lymph nodes can be identified as signal dropout on appropriate T2*-weighted sequences. Lymph nodes and lymph node regions that are occupied by metastatic tumor, however, lose their reticuloendothelial system function and, thus, do not exhibit the appropriate signal loss on T2*-weighted series.

The USPIO agent Combidex (Advanced Magnetic, Cambridge, Massachusetts) is approved for use in humans in Europe and is currently in clinical trials in the United States. USPIO-enhanced imaging has been shown to stage nodal spread of disease accurately in a variety of pelvic malignancies including cervical and bladder cancer [53,54]. In prostate cancer, USPIO particles can predict the presence of lymph node metastatic disease including micrometastatic disease [55]. Additional studies (including multisite trials) are required to further evaluate the potential role of USPIO nodal imaging in evaluating prostate cancer patients.

Post therapy/recurrence

Following curative therapy by surgery or radiation therapy, patients are generally monitored by serial PSA testing. A post-therapy PSA nadir followed by detectable or rising PSA is a strong predictor of disease recurrence. Regional lymph node recurrence can generally be depicted by CT scan and osseous metastases by bone scan. If disseminated metastatic disease is excluded, then the tumor may be locally recurrent.

MR imaging can be used to document the extent of locally recurrent disease. After radical prostatectomy, endorectal coil MR imaging is sensitive for detecting tumor nodules in the prostatectomy bed and adjacent tissue [56,57].

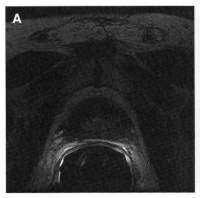 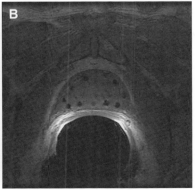

Fig. 9. Radiation changes in the prostate. (*A*) Axial T2W image with endorectal coil reveals a small prostate gland. There is uniform dark signal on T2W imaging, with little differentiation between PZ and central gland. (*B*) Axial T1W gradient echo image at same location demonstrates signal voids within the PZ, representing radiation seeds.

After radiation therapy, the irradiated prostate atrophies and appears shrunken, with low T2W signal intensity (Fig. 9) [58]. MR imaging is less useful in detecting intraprostatic recurrence when there is rise in PSA after radiation treatment because the contrast between intraprostatic tumor recurrence and adjacent prostate tissue may be low. In the setting of radiation-induced metabolic atrophy, however, MRSI has been shown to identify local recurrence [59,60].

Summary

Currently, endorectal coil MR imaging has the ability to improve accuracy in staging of localized prostate cancer. The addition of MRSI has further improved the sensitivity of MR imaging for intraprostatic tumor localization. Additional refinements and techniques are expected to further improve the performance of MR imaging for prostate cancer imaging and to aid in patient management. Further studies are required to identify the ideal role for MR imaging in the diagnosis and management of prostate cancer.

References

[1] American Cancer Society. Cancer facts and figures 2005. Atlanta (GA): American Cancer Society; 2005.

[2] Potosky AL, Miller BA, Albertsen PC, et al. The role of increasing detection in the rising incidence of prostate cancer. JAMA 1995;273:548–52.

[3] Roberts RO, Bergstralh EJ, Katusic SK, et al. Decline in prostate cancer mortality from 1980 to 1997, and an update on incidence trends in Olmsted County, Minnesota. J Urol 1999;161: 529–33.

[4] Moul JW, Wu H, Sun L, et al. Epidemiology of radical prostatectomy for localized prostate cancer in the era of prostate-specific antigen: an overview of the Department of Defense Center for Prostate Disease Research national database. Surgery 2002;132:213–9.

[5] Etzioni R, Penson DF, Legler JM, et al. Overdiagnosis due to prostate-specific antigen screening: lessons from US prostate cancer incidence trends. J Natl Cancer Inst 2002;94:981–90.

[6] Schnall MD, Lenkinski RE, Pollack HM, et al. Prostate: MR imaging with an endorectal surface coil. Radiology 1989;172:570–4.

[7] Perrotti M, Han KR, Epstein RE, et al. Prospective evaluation of endorectal magnetic resonance imaging to detect tumor foci in men with prior negative prostatic biopsy: a pilot study. J Urol 1999;162:1314–7.

[8] Beyersdorff D, Taupitz M, Winkelmann B, et al. Patients with a history of elevated prostate-specific antigen levels and negative transrectal US-guided quadrant or sextant biopsy results: value of MR imaging. Radiology 2002;224:701–6.

[9] Saigal CS, Pashos CL, Henning JM, et al. Variations in use of imaging in a national sample of men with early-stage prostate cancer. Urology 2002;59:400–4.

[10] Liney GP, Turnbull LW, Knowles AJ. A simple method for the correction of endorectal surface coil inhomogeneity in prostate imaging. J Magn Reson Imaging 1998;8:994–7.

[11] White S, Hricak H, Forstner R, et al. Prostate cancer: effect of postbiopsy hemorrhage on interpretation of MR images. Radiology 1995;195:385–90.

[12] Coakley FV, Kurhanewicz J, Lu Y, et al. Prostate cancer tumor volume: measurement with endorectal MR and MR spectroscopic imaging. Radiology 2002;223:91–7.

[13] Blute ML, Bergstralh EJ, Iocca A, et al. Use of Gleason score, prostate specific antigen, seminal vesicle and margin status to predict biochemical failure after radical prostatectomy. J Urol 2001; 165:119–25.

[14] Han M, Partin AW, Zahurak M, et al. Biochemical (prostate specific antigen) recurrence probability following radical prostatectomy for clinically localized prostate cancer. J Urol 2003; 169:517–23.

[15] Schellhammer PF. Radical prostatectomy. Patterns of local failure and survival in 67 patients. Urology 1988;31:191–7.

[16] Partin AW, Yoo J, Carter HB, et al. The use of prostate specific antigen, clinical stage and Gleason score to predict pathological stage in men with localized prostate cancer. J Urol 1993;150:110–4.

[17] D'Amico AV, Whittington R, Schnall M, et al. The impact of the inclusion of endorectal coil magnetic resonance imaging in a multivariate analysis to predict clinically unsuspected extraprostatic cancer. Cancer 1995;75:2368–72.

[18] Langlotz CP, Schnall MD, Malkowicz SB, et al. Cost-effectiveness of endorectal magnetic resonance imaging for the staging of prostate cancer. Acad Radiol 1996;3(Suppl 1):S24–7.

[19] Langlotz C, Schnall M, Pollack H. Staging of prostatic cancer: accuracy of MR imaging. Radiology 1995;194:645–6 [discussion: 647–8].

[20] D'Amico AV. The role of MR imaging in the selection of therapy for prostate cancer. Magn Reson Imaging Clin N Am 1996;4:471–9.

[21] Hricak H, Wang L, Wei DC, et al. The role of preoperative endorectal magnetic resonance imaging in the decision regarding whether to preserve or resect neurovascular bundles during radical retropubic prostatectomy. Cancer 2004; 100:2655–63.

[22] Yu KK, Hricak H. Imaging prostate cancer. Radiol Clin North Am 2000;38:59–85 [viii].

[23] Kurhanewicz J, Vigneron DB, Hricak H, et al. Three-dimensional H-1 MR spectroscopic imaging of the in situ human prostate with high (0.24–0.7-cm3) spatial resolution. Radiology 1996; 198:795–805.

[24] Wang L, Hricak H, Kattan MW, et al. Prediction of organ-confined prostate cancer: incremental value of MR imaging and MR spectroscopic imaging to staging nomograms. Radiology 2006; 238:597–603.

[25] Futterer JJ, Scheenen TW, Huisman HJ, et al. Initial experience of 3 tesla endorectal coil magnetic resonance imaging and 1H-spectroscopic imaging of the prostate. Invest Radiol 2004;39: 671–80.

[26] Bloch BN, Rofsky NM, Baroni RH, et al. 3 Tesla magnetic resonance imaging of the prostate with combined pelvic phased-array and endorectal coils: initial experience (1). Acad Radiol 2004;11:863–7.

[27] De Meerleer G, Villeirs G, Bral S, et al. The magnetic resonance detected intraprostatic lesion in prostate cancer: planning and delivery of intensity-modulated radiotherapy. Radiother Oncol 2005;75:325–33.

[28] Buyyounouski MK, Horwitz EM, Price RA, et al. Intensity-modulated radiotherapy with MRI simulation to reduce doses received by erectile tissue during prostate cancer treatment. Int J Radiat Oncol Biol Phys 2004;58:743–9.

[29] Debois M, Oyen R, Maes F, et al. The contribution of magnetic resonance imaging to the three-dimensional treatment planning of localized prostate cancer. Int J Radiat Oncol Biol Phys 1999;45:857–65.

[30] DiBiase SJ, Hosseinzadeh K, Gullapalli RP, et al. Magnetic resonance spectroscopic imaging-guided brachytherapy for localized prostate cancer. Int J Radiat Oncol Biol Phys 2002;52: 429–38.

[31] Zaider M, Zelefsky MJ, Lee EK, et al. Treatment planning for prostate implants using magnetic-resonance spectroscopy imaging. Int J Radiat Oncol Biol Phys 2000;47:1085–96.

[32] Mizowaki T, Cohen GN, Fung AY, et al. Towards integrating functional imaging in the treatment of prostate cancer with radiation: the registration of the MR spectroscopy imaging to ultrasound/ CT images and its implementation in treatment planning. Int J Radiat Oncol Biol Phys 2002; 54:1558–64.

[33] Huisman HJ, Futterer JJ, van Lin EN, et al. Prostate cancer: precision of integrating functional MR imaging with radiation therapy treatment by using fiducial gold markers. Radiology 2005; 236:311–7.

[34] Hirose M, Bharatha A, Hata N, et al. Quantitative MR imaging assessment of prostate gland deformation before and during MR imaging-guided brachytherapy. Acad Radiol 2002;9:906–12.

[35] Atalar E, Menard C. MR-guided interventions for prostate cancer. Magn Reson Imaging Clin N Am 2005;13:491–504.

[36] Susil RC, Camphausen K, Choyke P, et al. System for prostate brachytherapy and biopsy in a standard 1.5 T MRI scanner. Magn Reson Med 2004; 52:683–7.

[37] Menard C, Susil RC, Choyke P, et al. MRI-guided HDR prostate brachytherapy in standard 1.5T scanner. Int J Radiat Oncol Biol Phys 2004;59: 1414–23.

[38] D'Amico AV, Cormack RA, Tempany CM. MRI-guided diagnosis and treatment of prostate cancer. N Engl J Med 2001;344:776–7.

[39] D'Amico AV, Cormack R, Tempany CM, et al. Real-time magnetic resonance image-guided interstitial brachytherapy in the treatment of select patients with clinically localized prostate cancer. Int J Radiat Oncol Biol Phys 1998;42: 507–15.

[40] Cormack RA, Kooy H, Tempany CM, et al. A clinical method for real-time dosimetric guidance of transperineal 125I prostate implants using interventional magnetic resonance imaging. Int J Radiat Oncol Biol Phys 2000;46:207–14.

[41] Kaplan I, Oldenburg NE, Meskell P, et al. Real time MRI-ultrasound image guided stereotactic prostate biopsy. Magn Reson Imaging 2002;20: 295–9.

[42] Huch Boni RA, Boner JA, Lutolf UM, et al. Contrast-enhanced endorectal coil MRI in local staging of prostate carcinoma. J Comput Assist Tomogr 1995;19:232–7.

[43] Noworolski SM, Henry RG, Vigneron DB, et al. Dynamic contrast-enhanced MRI in normal and abnormal prostate tissues as defined by biopsy, MRI, and 3D MRSI. Magn Reson Med 2005;53: 249–55.

[44] Buckley DL, Roberts C, Parker GJ, et al. Prostate cancer: evaluation of vascular characteristics with dynamic contrast-enhanced T1-weighted MR imaging—initial experience. Radiology 2004; 233:709–15.

[45] Padhani AR, Gapinski CJ, Macvicar DA, et al. Dynamic contrast enhanced MRI of prostate cancer: correlation with morphology and tumour stage, histological grade and PSA. Clin Radiol 2000;55:99–109.

[46] Schlemmer HP, Merkle J, Grobholz R, et al. Can pre-operative contrast-enhanced dynamic MR imaging for prostate cancer predict microvessel density in prostatectomy specimens? Eur Radiol 2004;14:309–17.

[47] Engelbrecht MR, Huisman HJ, Laheij RJ, et al. Discrimination of prostate cancer from normal peripheral zone and central gland tissue by using dynamic contrast-enhanced MR imaging. Radiology 2003;229:248–54.

[48] Futterer JJ, Engelbrecht MR, Huisman HJ, et al. Staging prostate cancer with dynamic contrast-enhanced endorectal MR imaging prior to radical prostatectomy: experienced versus less experienced readers. Radiology 2005;237:541–9.

[49] Shimofusa R, Fujimoto H, Akamata H, et al. Diffusion-weighted imaging of prostate cancer. J Comput Assist Tomogr 2005;29:149–53.

[50] Sato C, Naganawa S, Nakamura T, et al. Differentiation of noncancerous tissue and cancer lesions by apparent diffusion coefficient values

in transition and peripheral zones of the prostate. J Magn Reson Imaging 2005;21:258–62.

[51] Hosseinzadeh K, Schwarz SD. Endorectal diffusion-weighted imaging in prostate cancer to differentiate malignant and benign peripheral zone tissue. J Magn Reson Imaging 2004;20:654–61.

[52] van Dorsten FA, van der Graaf M, Engelbrecht MR, et al. Combined quantitative dynamic contrast-enhanced MR imaging and (1)H MR spectroscopic imaging of human prostate cancer. J Magn Reson Imaging 2004;20:279–87.

[53] Rockall AG, Sohaib SA, Harisinghani MG, et al. Diagnostic performance of nanoparticle-enhanced magnetic resonance imaging in the diagnosis of lymph node metastases in patients with endometrial and cervical cancer. J Clin Oncol 2005;23:2813–21.

[54] Deserno WM, Harisinghani MG, Taupitz M, et al. Urinary bladder cancer: preoperative nodal staging with ferumoxtran-10-enhanced MR imaging. Radiology 2004;233:449–56.

[55] Harisinghani MG, Barentsz J, Hahn PF, et al. Noninvasive detection of clinically occult lymph-node metastases in prostate cancer. N Engl J Med 2003;348:2491–9.

[56] Sella T, Schwartz LH, Swindle PW, et al. Suspected local recurrence after radical prostatectomy: endorectal coil MR imaging. Radiology 2004;231:379–85.

[57] Silverman JM, Krebs TL. MR imaging evaluation with a transrectal surface coil of local recurrence of prostatic cancer in men who have undergone radical prostatectomy. AJR Am J Roentgenol 1997;168:379–85.

[58] Chan TW, Kressel HY. Prostate and seminal vesicles after irradiation: MR appearance. J Magn Reson Imaging 1991;1:503–11.

[59] Pucar D, Shukla-Dave A, Hricak H, et al. Prostate cancer: correlation of MR imaging and MR spectroscopy with pathologic findings after radiation therapy-initial experience. Radiology 2005;236:545–53.

[60] Coakley FV, Teh HS, Qayyum A, et al. Endorectal MR imaging and MR spectroscopic imaging for locally recurrent prostate cancer after external beam radiation therapy: preliminary experience. Radiology 2004;233:441–8.

ELSEVIER
SAUNDERS

RADIOLOGIC
CLINICS
OF NORTH AMERICA

Radiol Clin N Am 44 (2006) 735–748

Image-Guided Brachytherapy for Prostate Cancer

Deborah J. Rubens, MD[a],*, Yan Yu, PhD[b],
Agnieszka Szot Barnes, MD[c], John G. Strang, MD[a],
Ralph Brasacchio, MD[b]

- Low dose rate brachytherapy: ultrasound guidance
- MR-guided permanent prostate brachytherapy: experience from the Brigham and Women's Hospital
- Summary
- References

Prostate cancer is the most common cancer after skin cancer in United States men and the second most common cause of cancer death, with an expected incidence of 230,090 in 2005 and an estimated 30,350 deaths [1]. The incidence of prostate cancer has risen in part because the average life expectancy has increased. Additional cases are being diagnosed due to prostate-specific antigen (PSA) screening. This PSA-detected cancer is more frequently early-stage disease, which is moderately differentiated and confined to the prostate [2]. The time-honored curative therapy for localized prostate carcinoma is surgery (radical prostatectomy). Nonprogression is defined as a stable low or undetectable serum PSA. The nonprogression rate of radical prostatectomy has been reported in several large series and ranges from 76% to 80% at 5 years, 68% to 81% at 7 years, and 68% to 71% at 10 years [3]. In addition to PSA-defined failures to cure, surgery has immediate and long-term complications. Short-term complications include those from anesthesia and blood loss or infection following the surgery. Long-term complications are primarily impotence or incontinence. Thus, alternatives to surgery have been sought.

The most common alternative initially was external beam radiation therapy (EBRT). Radiation treats not only the prostate but also the periprostatic tissues and can include the regional lymph nodes. In a large retrospective study of 59,876 cancer registrants with varying pathologic tumor grade, EBRT had a slightly poorer prostate cancer–specific survival compared with surgery [4]. Prostatectomy yielded 10-year prostate cancer–specific survival of 94% for low-grade tumors (Gleason score 2–4), 87% for moderate-grade tumors (Gleason score 5–7), and 67% for high-grade tumors (Gleason score 8–10). Radiation therapy yielded 90%, 76%, and 53% 10-year prostate cancer–specific survival rates in comparable groups. An advantage of one treatment over another is difficult to ascertain from this study, however, because patients were

[a] Department of Imaging Sciences, University of Rochester Medical Center, Box 648, 601 Elmwood Avenue, Rochester, NY 14642, USA
[b] Department of Radiation Oncology, University of Rochester Medical Center, Box 648, 601 Elmwood Avenue, Rochester, NY 14642, USA
[c] Radiology-Brigham and Women's Hospital, 75 Francis Street, Boston, MA 02115, USA
* Corresponding author.
E-mail address: deborah_rubens@urmc.rochester.edu (D.J. Rubens).

doi:10.1016/j.rcl.2006.07.006

not randomized regarding treatment decisions or stratified for risk factors that might have biased the outcomes [4]. The slight differences in radiation effectiveness versus surgery for cure may be offset by better patient tolerance for radiotherapy. Outcomes comparing radical prostatectomy versus EBRT showed higher rates of incontinence (9.6% versus 3.5%), impotence (79.6% versus 61.5%), and urinary stricture requiring treatment (17.4% versus 7.2%) in patients who had surgery. Patients who underwent EBRT, however, had higher rates of proctitis (18.7% versus 1.6%) [5]. As a result of this trade-off, EBRT has generally been chosen as therapy for prostate cancer patients unable to tolerate surgery, for patients older than 65 years, and for treatment of advanced disease that has spread beyond the prostate. Unlike surgery, which ideally removes the cancer all at one time, radiation primarily kills only the cancer cells that are dividing. Because prostate cancer has a long doubling time, the response to radiation takes place over the course of months or years. The time commitment of an approximately 8-week radiation course and the side effects from radiation to the adjacent bladder and rectum are detractors from EBRT. Thus, alternative forms of radiation therapy were sought.

"Brachytherapy" is derived from the Greek word *brachio*, which means short. In brachytherapy, the path from the radiation source to the tissue target is short, which minimizes unwanted side effects to the surrounding structures and minimizes motion of the target, permitting a more tightly confined radiation field. Historically, brachytherapy was first described in the 1900s using radium needles and a transperineal approach [6]. The advent of permanent iodine seeds in the 1960s permitted an open "free-hand" retropubic approach, but it was technically unsatisfactory due to poor dosimetry and higher recurrence rates than EBRT or radical prostatectomy.

There are currently two forms of brachytherapy: high dose rate (HDR) and low dose rate (LDR). LDR or permanent implant brachytherapy is far more common and places radioactive seeds directly into the prostate to deliver the radiation dose directly to the gland. Modern LDR brachytherapy developed in the 1980s with the advent of real-time transrectal ultrasound (TRUS) guidance, which permitted direct visualization of the needles and seeds in relation to the prostatic tissue. A permanent implant can also be performed with CT but the ultrasound approach was easily learned by urologists and became the standard of care. CT is now largely used to calculate postimplantation dosimetry. MR imaging can also be used for LDR brachytherapy and has the advantage of better three-dimensional

visualization of the prostate margins and potentially better visualization of the prostate cancer. These advantages, however, may be offset by the increased cost of MR imaging compared with TRUS, increased procedure time, and lack of widespread availability of interventional MR imaging facilities.

To plan seed placement, the size and shape of the prostate must be known so that an appropriate tumoricidal dose can be delivered. Ultrasound, CT, or MR imaging is used to plan the procedure. One of two radioactive sources is commonly used in the radioactive seeds: palladium 103 or iodine 125. Palladium has a half-life of 17 days and emits 21 keV mean photon energy, whereas iodine has a half-life of 59 days but emits 27 keV. The more energetic iodine 125 theoretically travels further in the body. Because of the shorter half-life, palladium implants generally require more seeds of higher-unit strengths to deliver an adequate dose to the prostate but are thought to deliver less radiation to the adjacent rectum and bladder [6]. Because the seeds remain permanently within the patient, gland swelling during the procedure or seed migration along the needle track may alter the actual dose from the original planned dose. One solution to this is better control of the radiation source over a shorter period of time.

HDR brachytherapy developed in the early 1990s using iridium 192, which emits 400 keV and requires only 10 to 15 minutes to deliver a therapeutic dose to a localized region [7]. In HDR, multiple needles are placed intraoperatively within the prostate, cystoscopy is performed to exclude needle penetration of the bladder mucosa, the needles are sutured in place, and a three-dimensional treatment plan is performed with the needles in place using ultrasound or CT, depending on the institution [8]. The patient is transferred to a shielded treatment area where the iridium source is then placed into one needle at a time using a robotic afterloader. The robot places the radioactive source for a variable amount of time in each position throughout the needle. This controls the location and dwell time of the source to deliver a precise amount of radiation to each portion of the gland while sparing the bladder, urethra, and rectum. This procedure is repeated for each tube until the entire prostate has received a certain prescribed dose. For HDR, the total dose to the entire prostate is delivered in multiple fractions, separated by at least 6 hours. Some institutions use as few as two fractions separated by 6 or more hours, whereas others use up to four fractions, which may be within 24 hours or separated by several days. At the conclusion of all the fractions, the source and tubes are removed. Although preliminary results from HDR implants are promising, the number of patients treated is far less than with LDR (the current standard of care). Compared with EBRT, the patient appeal of LDR or HDR brachytherapy is a 1-day outpatient procedure (LDR) or a 2-day procedure with one night in the hospital (HDR) instead of an 8-week, daily treatment regimen.

Low dose rate brachytherapy: ultrasound guidance

Who should undergo brachytherapy? In 1999, the American Brachytherapy Society (ABS) published recommendations for permanent implant brachytherapy [9]. The ABS recommends LDR brachytherapy alone (so-called "monotherapy") for patients who have a high likelihood of organ-confined disease as defined by preoperative staging according to the American Joint Committee on Cancer (Box 1) [10]. Patient inclusion criteria also includes a life expectancy of at least 5 years and no large transurethral prostatectomy defects, unacceptable operative risks, or known distant metastases. Monotherapy is recommended for patients who have tumor stage T1c to T2a disease with a pathologic Gleason score of 6 or less and a serum PSA of less than 10 ng/mL. Patients who have a Gleason score of 7, stage T2b disease, or a PSA between 10 and 20 ng/mL are recommended to be treated with monotherapy or with brachytherapy combined with EBRT or hormonal therapy. The authors' institution currently follows these guidelines, individualizing therapy for the patients who fall between the definite monotherapy and the combined therapy criteria. For patients who have stage T2c and higher, Gleason scores of 8 to 10, or PSA levels greater than 20 ng/mL, the ABS recommends combined EBRT and brachytherapy. In patients who have glands greater than 60 mL, the ABS recommends that hormonal therapy should be considered to shrink the gland before brachytherapy.

When patients meet eligibility criteria for brachytherapy, they are referred to ultrasound for a volumetric study to determine whether there is potential pubic arch interference with needle placement and whether they have an enlarged gland. Either of these situations would result in a recommendation for hormone therapy to shrink the prostate before implantation. The pubic arch may physically obstruct the transperineal needle access to the anterior and lateral portions of the prostate, making it difficult or impossible to implant seeds in these locations. If this restriction exists, the implantation may be modified by angling the template and ultrasound probe to achieve better needle access; however, the ability to correct this problem is limited by a maximum of about 10° to

15° of angulation at most. Severe pubic arch interference is considered a contraindication to performing the implant.

Both CT and TRUS have been used to detect pubic arch interference. In the CT-based technique, the largest extent of the prostate is graphically marked onto the axial slice containing the pubic arch. If significant overlap exists between the two structures, then pubic arch interference is likely to be encountered. A shortcoming of this technique is that the patient is not in the dorsal lithotomy position during the CT study, so the relationship between the prostate and the pubic arch is different than during actual implantation.

Prostate ultrasound is performed in the dorsal lithotomy position using a cradle fixed to the table. The cradle holds the TRUS transducer and manually steps it in a cranial-caudal direction at 5-mm increments. Patients are scanned at as high a transducer frequency as possible, from 5 to 7 MHz, depending on gland size and attenuation. The ultrasound probe is first moved to an axial slice on which the pubic bone–soft tissue interface is visible as an echogenic interface with acoustic shadowing beyond it (Fig. 1). The location of the pubic arch is traced on the ultrasound screen as a graphic overlay that persists in sequential images. The probe is then moved in a cranial-caudal direction to visualize the entire prostate on successive axial slices, with the tracing of the pubic arch overlaid on the images (see Fig. 1). Pubic arch interference is defined as any prostate tissue that projects beyond the outline of the arch, whether anterior (Fig. 2), lateral (Fig. 3), or both. The advantages of this technique are that it can be combined with a prostate volume study and it is performed with the patient in the treatment position [11]. Preimplant volumetric planning is recommended by the ABS for all patients [9] and consists of tracing the outline of the gland on each axial slice where prostate tissue is visualized (Fig. 4). These tracings are transferred to a treatment planning program to determine the appropriate placement of seeds and the number of seeds and specific seed strength that need to be ordered to deliver the required radiation dose.

The location of the seeds is distributed to give an adequate dose to the prostate while sparing the centrally located urethra and the adjacent posterior rectal wall. Reducing the central dose relative to the periphery is important because of potential urinary complications from a high urethral dose. Accordingly, the ABS recommends that a modified peripheral dosimetry method be used for prostate implants and that urethral dose is carefully examined in an effort to minimize the length of urethra receiving greater than 200% of the prescribed dose [9]. For monotherapy, the ABS recommends that

---

Box 1: Prostate cancer staging: TNM method adapted from the American Joint Committee on Cancer

Primary tumor (T)
TX: Primary tumor cannot be assessed
T0: No evidence of primary tumor
T1: Clinically inapparent tumor not palpable nor visible by imaging
T1a: Tumor incidental histologic finding in ≤5% of tissue resected
T1b: Tumor incidental histologic finding in >5% of tissue resected
T2: Tumor confined within prostate
T2a: Tumor involves 50% of ≤1 lobe or less
T2b: Tumor involves >50% of 1 lobe but not both lobes
T1c: Tumor identified by needle biopsy (eg, because of elevated PSA)
T2c: Tumor involves both lobes
T3: Tumor extends through the prostate capsule
T3a: Extracapsular extension (unilateral or bilateral)
T3b: Tumor invades seminal vesicle(s)
T4: Tumor is fixed or invades adjacent structures other than seminal vesicles: bladder neck, external
    sphincter, rectum, levator muscles, and/or pelvic wall

Regional lymph nodes (N)
Regional lymph nodes are the nodes of the true pelvis and distant lymph nodes are outside the true
pelvis
NX: Regional lymph nodes were not assessed
N0: No regional lymph node metastasis

Distant metastasis (M)[a]
MX: Distant metastasis cannot be assessed (not evaluated by any modality)
M0: No distant metastasis
M1: Distant metastasis
M1a: Nonregional lymph node(s)
M1b: Bone(s)
M1c: Other site(s) with or without bone disease

Histopathologic grade (G)
GX: Grade cannot be assessed
G1: Well differentiated (slight anaplasia) (Gleason grade 2–4)
G2: Moderately differentiated (moderate anaplasia) (Gleason grade 5–6)
G3–4: Poorly differentiated or undifferentiated (marked anaplasia) (Gleason grade 7–10)

American Joint Committee on Cancer stage groupings
Stage I: T1a, N0, M0, G1
Stage II: T1a, N0, M0, G2–4
        T1b, N0, M0, any G
        T1c, N0, M0, any G
        T1, N0, M0, any G
        T2, N0, M0, any G
Stage III: T3, N0, M0, any G
Stage IV: T4, N0, M0, any G
        Any T, N1, M0, any G
        Any T, any N, M1, any G

[a] When more than one site of metastasis is present, the most advanced category (pM1c) is used.
Used with permission of the American Joint Committee on Cancer (AJCC), Chicago, Illinois. The original source for this material is the AJCC Cancer Staging Manual, 6th edition. New York: Springer; 2002. Available at: www.springeronline.com.

---

patients receive a dose of 115 to 120 Gy for palladium 103 implants and 144 Gy (American Association of Physics and Medicine Task Group 43) for iodine 125 implants [9].

After preplanning is performed and the choice of seed type is made by the radiation oncologist, the patient is scheduled for the operating room or outpatient surgery suite, depending on the institution. Anesthesia is delivered by way of a spinal or with general anesthesia, depending on surgeon and patient preference. The bowel is prepared with an enema to reduce air and stool interference for TRUS. When brachytherapy programs were first initiated, the procedure began as patients were

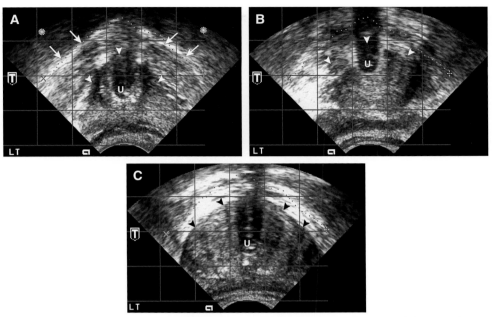

Fig. 1. Finding and tracing the pubic arch with ultrasound. (*A*) Axial image at the level of the apex demonstrates an echogenic interface (*arrows*) with shadowing anterior to it (*asterisks*). The arch is traced with a dotted line. The prostate anterior margin is denoted by arrowheads. This patient has a Foley catheter in the urethra (U). (*B, C*) The arch tracing remains on each image as sequential images are obtained from the base (*B*) through the midgland (*C*) and back to the apex (*A*).

placed into dorsolithotomy position, as close as possible to the preplan position. Needles were then placed according to the initial volumetric ultrasound plan. It was soon recognized, however, that patient position could change significantly between the initial plan and surgery and that a different orientation of the irregularly shaped prostate could lead to needle and seed placement beyond the confines of the prostate or inaccurately within the prostate. This incorrect needle placement could result in underdosing of the target organ or overdosing of the target or critical structures such as the urethra or rectum. In addition, if the patient had received hormonal therapy or EBRT before the implant, then substantial changes in gland volume occurred between preplanning and treatment. Therefore, the ABS recently recommended that intraoperative dosimetry planning be performed to achieve the intended dose to the appropriate areas [12,13]. At the University of Rochester Medical Center, the authors use a locally developed prostate implant planning engine for radiotherapy (PIPER) [14]. To begin intraoperative planning, the TRUS probe is aligned with the long axis of the prostate (parallel to the urethra), and the ultrasound probe and needle template are secured within the stepper device and attached to the operating table (Fig. 5). Three needles are then placed through the template into the prostate: one on the right anterolateral, one

on the left anterolateral, and one posterior between the urethra and the rectum in the midline (Fig. 6). These three needles serve to stabilize the gland and to align the prostate with the treatment plan that will subsequently be derived. The prostate is imaged axially in 5-mm increments from the base to the apex, and images are transferred from the ultrasound machine to the PIPER computer. There the images are traced by the radiologist to delineate the outline of the prostate, the urethra, and the anterior rectal margin using an automated segmentation algorithm that requires placing only a few points on each structure to develop the contour (see Fig. 6). Dosimetric planning is performed using the inverse planning engine (or optimization). This evaluation is a continuous, automated interactive process of isodose review, dose volume histogram analysis, and assessment of the feasibility of the needle placement plan (eg, avoiding the urethra) during the actual procedure. A treatment plan is derived and approved by the radiation oncologist and radiation physicist (Fig. 7). The needles used for seed placement are then inserted into the prostate in the positions prescribed, with craniocaudal, mediolateral, and anteroposterior location of each needle confirmed by real-time ultrasound.

When the needles are in place, seed deployment begins. The authors use a Mick applicator (Mick

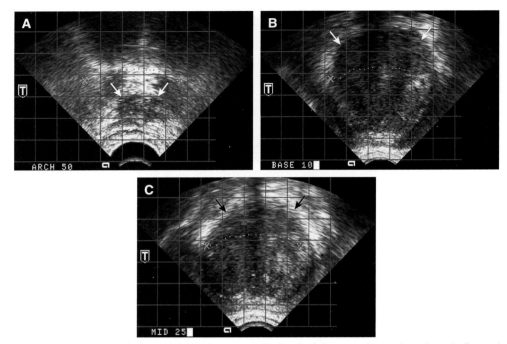

Fig. 2. Severe pubic arch interference. (*A*) Axial image at the level of the apex shows the relatively flat arch (*dotted line*) anterior to the prostate apex (*arrows*). Grid markers are spaced at 1-cm intervals. (*B*) Axial image at the base 4 cm cranial to position in (*A*) shows the position of the arch (*dotted line*) superimposed over the prostate (*arrows*). Almost 2 cm of tissue projects anterior to the position of the arch. (*C*) Axial image at the midgland shows persistant arch interference (the dotted line denotes arch position) with at least 30% of the gland inaccessible for implantation.

Radionuclear Instruments, Inc., Mount Vernon, New York), which loads the seeds into the prostate from prepackaged sterilized cartridges. Palladium or iodine seeds can be delivered in this way. Cartridges are kept in a shielded container to minimize exposure to operating room personnel. The number of seeds used in each needle can be adjusted, as determined clinically. For example, if there is gland swelling or if a needle cannot be placed in the exact location dictated by the plan, then seeds can be omitted or added. The total time for the procedure

including intraoperative planning, needle placement, and seed deployment ranges from 1 to 1.5 hours. Other brachytherapy groups use preloaded needles. When this method is selected, the seeds are loaded into a sterilized needle according to the preoperative plan and interspersed with biodegradable spacers. There is usually 5 mm of dead space at the needle tip that is sealed by a piece of bone wax or other sealant to prevent the seeds from exiting the needle during introduction into the prostate. The radioactive needle is then placed

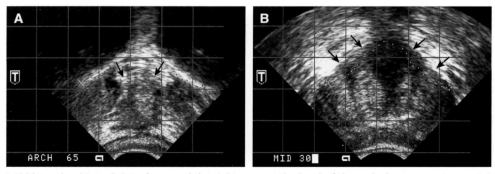

Fig. 3. Mild lateral pubic arch interference. (*A*) Axial image at the level of the arch shows a narrow arch (*dotted line*) well anterior to the prostate apex (*arrows*). (*B*) At the midgland level, the arch tracing (*dotted line*) overlaps the lateral anterior margins of the prostate on both sides (*arrows*).

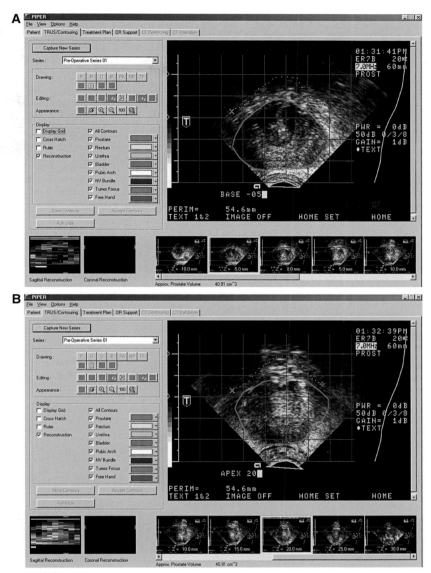

Fig. 4. Preoperative volume assessment. Selected axial images obtained sequentially from the base (*A*) to the apex (*B*) of the prostate after initial localization of the pubic arch (*dotted line*). Prostate margin is outlined in pink and rectal mucosa is traced in yellow. Images are numbered from position −10.0 to 30.0 of the stepper device and obtained in 5-mm increments, as shown on the horizontal strip below the selected image. Nine images were obtained in this patient; the second and seventh images are displayed with their tracings. The overlying grid has 1-cm spacing.

into the prostate and the seeds and spacers pushed out with a stylet. Preloading the needles is more time-consuming than using the applicator, especially when intraoperative planning is also performed [12].

The ABS recommends that postoperative dosimetry be performed for each patient [9] to confirm the dose delivered and to provide feedback to the brachytherapy team for quality assurance. The current recommended method is CT. Because the

apex and the base of the prostate are often difficult to identify precisely on CT, there has been a discrepancy in the measured gland size when the treatment planning ultrasound and the post-implant CT are compared, with measured volumes on CT being 20% to 40% larger than the measured ultrasound volumes. In addition, the prostate may have significant postoperative edema. For these reasons, it is recommended that postoperative dosimetry be performed no

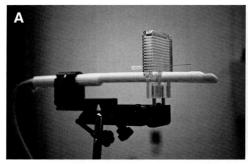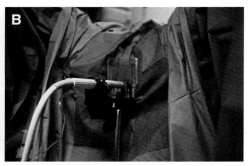

Fig. 5. Perineal template and ultrasound stepper device in place. (*A*) Photograph of the clear perineal template attached to the black metallic stepper device. The ultrasound transducer is held in a fixed position posterior to the clear template and can translate into and out of the patient and rotate from side to side. The template contains holes that accommodate 17- or 18-gauge needles spaced at 5 mm in each direction. The template is parallel to the patient's perineal skin and directs the needles from the perineum into the prostate in the caudal-to-cranial direction. A single needle is displayed. (*B*) Photograph of the patient's perineum with the transducer inserted into the rectum and the perineal template attached to the stepper device.

earlier than 4 weeks post implant [9]. The CT scan should include the entire prostate plus 2 cm above and below the gland to include any seeds that may be located there and to assess the position of the rectum and urethra to calculate the dose delivered to those organs [15]. The field of view should be reduced to include only the prostate and surrounding pelvis. Slices should be contiguous, and the slice thickness should be no greater than 5 mm, preferably 3 mm (Fig. 8) [15].

MR-guided permanent prostate brachytherapy: experience from the Brigham and Women's Hospital

The authors' eligibility criteria for MR-guided prostate brachytherapy include a clinical-stage assessment of T1cNXM0 (according to the American Joint Committee on Cancer), PSA level less than 10 ng/mL, biopsy Gleason score not greater than 7 out of 10, low cancer volumes, and an endorectal

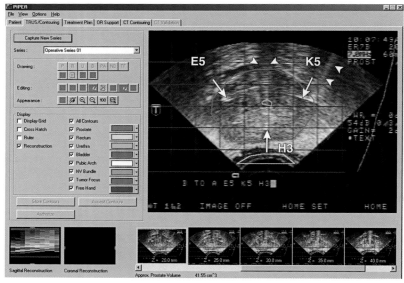

Fig. 6. Intraoperative localizer needles. Axial image of the prostate at the level of the base showing intraoperative treatment plan with echogenic localizing needles in place (*arrows*) inserted from positions E5, K5, and H3 on the external perineal grid. Note the reverberation artifact (*arrowheads*) that is also useful to identify needle position. Prostate margin is traced in pink, urethra is outlined in blue, and rectum in yellow. The treatment plan generated will label subsequent needle positions in relation to these initial three localizer needles, and the position of the seeds along the needles are identified with respect to the first axial slice at the base. The localizer needles help to stabilize the gland and may be implanted with seeds.

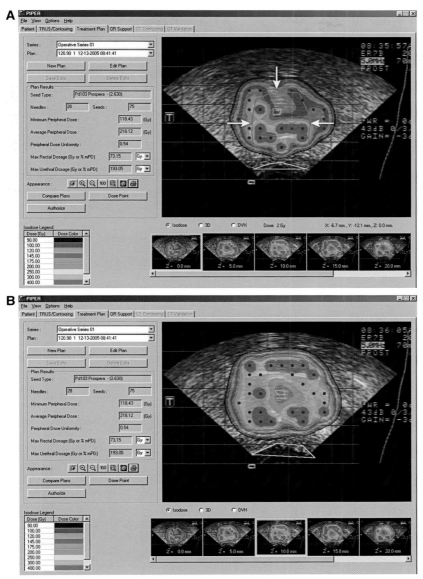

Fig. 7. Intraoperative plan. Axial images of the prostate at the base (*A*) and midgland (*B, C*) obtained sequentially at 5-mm intervals. The images in (*B*) and (*C*) are adjacent. Needle positions are displayed as blue dots, and needles containing seeds at that level are shown as red dots. Seeds are generally deposited at 10-mm intervals and, therefore, will not be displayed on adjacent slices, as exemplified by comparing images in (*B*) and (*C*). The prostate margin as originally traced on the intraoperative plan remains outlined in pink (*arrows*), the urethra in blue, and the rectum in yellow. The remaining colored regions represent the isodose delivered to each area of the prostate and to the surrounding tissues as indicated on the color code table in the lower left of each image. In this palladium implant, the minimum peripheral dose to the entire prostate is 118 Gy. As recommended by the ABS, the maximum urethral dose is less than 200% at 193 Gy, and the rectum is spared, with a maximum dose of 73 Gy.

coil 1.5-T MR imaging examination [16]. The authors do not use a volume cutoff in this program because pubic arch interference is not a problem with the transperineal MR-guided approach. The template can be moved, if necessary, at the end of needle placement to allow for angulation around the arch. Men who have had previous transurethral resection of the prostate are excluded.

All men have a 1.5-T endorectal coil MR imaging examination before the actual treatment. This examinaiton is done as part of the staging process to help exclude extraglandular disease, seminal vesicle

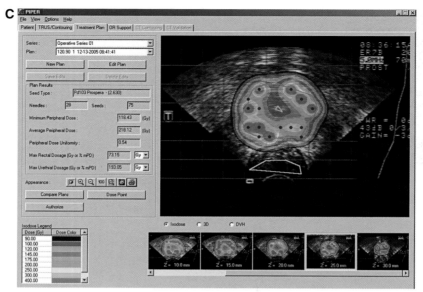

Fig. 7 (continued)

invasion, and possible spread to pelvic lymph nodes or bones. It also provides images for pretreatment planning and, when necessary, can be used in conjunction with "real-time" images acquired during the MR-guided brachytherapy procedure.

On the morning of the procedure, the patient comes to the suite after fasting the night before. For the actual procedure, the patient is positioned in an open configuration 0.5-T MR scanner (GE SIGNA MR Therapy System, General Electric, Milwaukee, Wisconsin) in the lithotomy position [17,18]. This MR unit was designed specially for interventional procedures by General Electric in December 1993. The SIGNA MR Therapy System consists of two annuli separated by about 60 cm, with the patient in a coaxial or radial position. The 30-cm diameter imaging volume operates at 0.5 T, with each of the individual magnets at 3.0 T. The SIGNA MR Therapy System has operator and remote consoles, with displays inside and outside the magnet opening for physician use during interventions. A complete integrated patient monitoring system is adjacent to the magnet in the shielded room. The open configuration of this scanner leaves a vertically oriented space for easy access to the patient (Fig. 9).

The patient enters the magnet awake and is positioned in lithotomy with the legs in MR-compatible boots. Initial imaging is performed with an external "wrap-around" coil to ensure the patient is correctly positioned. General anesthesia is induced and, with the anesthetized patient in position, a Foley catheter is inserted, the Plexiglas template for the needle

guidance is placed against the perineum and secured, and a rectal obturator is inserted.

The MR imaging is then performed. A series of T2-weighted images is acquired in the axial, coronal, and sagittal planes. These images, made without benefit of an endorectal coil at 0.5 T, are sufficient for recognizing the peripheral zone, the urethra, and rectum—all essential for treatment planning.

The MR images are analyzed and contoured by the radiologist, which is done by using the 0.5-T T2-weighted images alone or by registering or morphing them with T2-weighted images or spectroscopic results acquired previously with the endorectal coil at 1.5 T [19–21]. This morphing procedure is performed by an image processing team using three-dimensional Slicer software, a free, open-source software for two- and three-dimensional image display, registration, and segmentation of medical images (see www.slicer.org for more information). It allows for incorporating the high–spatial resolution, high-contrast images or spectroscopic data acquired previously at 1.5 T directly into the lower-contrast, lower-field strength images being acquired "real-time" during the procedure (Fig. 10). Using the T2-weighted 0.5-T images or the combination of morphed 1.5-T/0.5-T data, the brachytherapy team can (1) identify the peripheral zone as the clinical target volume and (2) identify structures to be avoided (like the rectal wall and urethra) for proper placement of the iodine 125 seeds. The depth of catheter insertion and number of iodine 125 seeds may then be calculated using

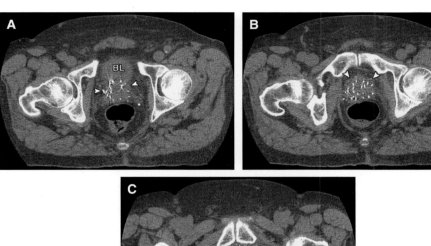

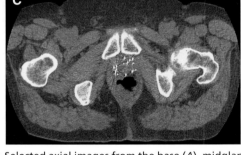

Fig. 8. Postoperative dosimetry. Selected axial images from the base (*A*), midgland (*B*), and apex (*C*) are obtained at 3-mm intervals with a small field of view. Prostate (*arrowheads*) is difficult to segment from the adjacent soft tissue, especially from the bladder (BL) at the base and from the urethra and perineal soft tissues at the apex. Seeds are very bright and some are noted on sequential slices. Because the seeds are 4 mm in length, they frequently appear on more than one CT slice, and should not be counted twice.

a software program developed in house by Cormack and Kooy and colleagues [22,23].

After the plan is developed, the set of needles (all 18-G E-Z-EM needles [E-Z-EM Inc., Westbury, New

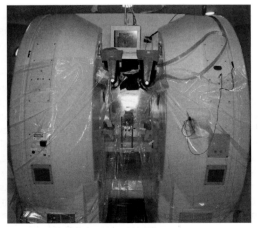

Fig. 9. Open 0.5-T MR system for performing image-guided procedures. *From* Barnes AS, Tempany CM. Image-guided minimally invasive therapy. In: Richie JP, D'Amico A, editors. Urologic Oncology. Philadelphia: Elsevier; 2005. p. 114; with permission.

York]) are preloaded with the iodine 125 radiation sources and the team of physicians begins the implant. Each needle is measured to the prescribed depth and inserted into the patient, transperineally, though the template. Following each catheter insertion, rapid gradient echo images are acquired in the axial plane to determine the position of the catheter (Fig. 11). The susceptibility-based T2* image contrast attained with gradient echo imaging makes the catheter appear as a well-defined black line whose location may be readily compared with the location sought in the treatment plan. The needle location undergoes an anatomic and dosimetric review. The radiologist can see the needle on the images and determine the trajectory, repositioning if it is off axis or misplaced. The dosimetric analysis is then performed. From the locations of the catheters in relation to the anatomy, dose volume histograms are calculated for the clinical target volume, anterior rectal wall, and urethra by medical physicists present during the procedure [23,24]. Adjustment of catheter positions is made until satisfactory dose volume histograms are achieved as agreed by the radiation oncologist and the team, at which point the seeds are deposited and catheters removed. The patient is taken to the recovery room and discharged home the following day.

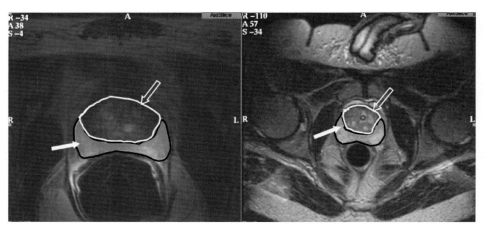

Fig. 10. Prostate gland segmentation and registration. Segmentation identifies peripheral zone (*solid arrow*) and central gland (*hollow arrow*) in pretherapy endorectal coil MR (1.5-T, *left image*) and MR-guided therapy images (0.5-T, *right image*). Registration matches the segmented areas in the different images. (*From* Barnes AS, Tempany CM. Image-guided minimally invasive therapy. In: Richie JP, D'Amico A, editors. Urologic Oncology. Philadelphia: Elsevier; 2005. p. 115; with permission.)

Approximately 6 weeks after the procedure, MR imaging and CT examinations of the prostate are performed to identify the location of the seeds and calculate final dose volume histograms. The CT images provide the most accurate visualization of seed locations, whereas the MR images better depict the underlying anatomy so that fusing the MR and CT images by way of image processing software allows for the best calculation of dose to the soft tissues in the vicinity of the seeds (Fig. 12).

The use of 1.5-T images and spectroscopic data in conjunction with real-time 0.5-T images acquired during the brachytherapy procedure requires intensive cooperation between physicians, image processing scientists, and medical physicists. Performing the spatial registration between endorectal coil–acquired images (in which the prostate is deformed somewhat by the endorectal coil) with images acquired without the endorectal coil at the lower field strength is a particularly vexing problem. Future strategies for improving MR-guided brachytherapy procedures are envisioned in which the seed placements can be performed in closed-bore 1.5-T or even 3-T units, facilitating the use of real-time high-quality images of the prostate and having the potential to use spectroscopic imaging methods [19,21] for improved targeting of the prostate carcinomas.

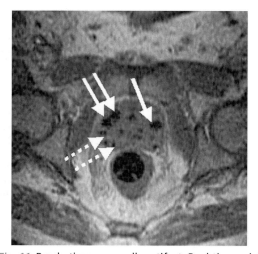

Fig. 11. Brachytherapy needle artifact. Real-time axial view of prostate gland on intra–MR-guided brachytherapy images. The solid arrows indicate the tips of the needles. The dashed arrows indicate locations of radioactive seeds.

Summary

Prostate brachytherapy offers an effective treatment for organ-confined prostate carcinoma. Compared with EBRT or surgery, it is rapidly delivered and well tolerated by patients, with minimal side effects. Volumetric imaging and image guidance play critical roles in patient selection, treatment planning, treatment delivery, and postimplant assessment. Costs, availability, and ease of use often dictate the local and regional differences in imaging approach, whether ultrasound, CT, or MR. Future volumetric image developments may permit multimodality image fusion to integrate tumor-specific imaging such as MR spectrospcopy or positron emission tomography/CT into real-time ultrasound, CT, or MR. We can expect many

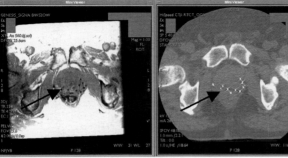

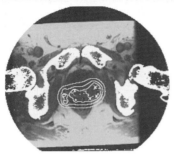

Fig. 12. MR-CT fusion of post–MR-guided brachytherapy images. Post-therapy MR image (*left*) and CT image (*middle*) are fused, resulting in an MR-CT image (*right*) to allow better visualization of individual seeds and facilitate dose-distribution calculation. Black arrows indicate radioactive seeds. (*From* Barnes AS, Tempany CM. Image-guided minimally invasive therapy. In: Richie JP, D'Amico A, editors. Urologic Oncology. Philadelphia: Elsevier; 2005. p. 121; with permission.)

improvements in image-guided prostate cancer therapy in the years to come.

References

[1] Jemal A, Murray T, Ward E, et al. Cancer statistics, 2005. CA Cancer J Clin 2005;55(1):10–30.

[2] Farkas A, Schneider D, Perrotti M, et al. National trends in the epidemiology of prostate cancer, 1973 to 1994: evidence for the effectiveness of prostate-specific antigen screening. Urology 1998;52:444–8.

[3] Perotti M, Gomella L. Treatment decisions: surgery versus brachytherapy. A urologist's perspective. In: Dicker A, Merrick G, Waterman F, et al, editors. Basic and advanced techniques in prostate brachytherapy. Abingdon, Oxfordshire, UK: Martin Dunitz Ltd.; 2005. p. 59–66.

[4] Lu-Yao GL, Yao S. Population-based study of long-term survival in patients with clinically localized prostate cancer. Lancet 1997;349:906–10.

[5] Potosky AL, Legler J, Alberson PC, et al. Health outcomes after prostatectomy or radiotherapy for prostate cancer: results from the Prostate Cancer Outcomes Study. J Natl Cancer Inst 2000;92:1582–92.

[6] Huynh N, Korman H. Brachytherapy from the urologist's perspective. In: Dicker A, Merrick G, Waterman F, et al, editors. Basic and advanced techniques in prostate brachytherapy. Abingdon, Oxfordshire, UK: Martin Dunitz Ltd.; 2005. p. 75–82.

[7] Badiozamani K, Mate T, Gottesman J. High dose rate 192Ir prostate brachytherapy. In: Dicker A, Merrick G, Waterman F, et al, editors. Basic and advanced techniques in prostate brachytherapy. Abingdon, Oxfordshire, UK: Martin Dunitz Ltd.; 2005. p. 295–302.

[8] Martinez A, Demanes J, Galale R, et al. High dose rate afterloading 192Ir prostate brachytherapy. In: Dicker A, Merrick G, Waterman F, et al, editors. Basic and advanced techniques in prostate brachytherapy. Abingdon, Oxfordshire, UK: Martin Dunitz Ltd.; 2005. p. 311–25.

[9] Nag S, Beyer D, Friedland J, et al. American Brachytherapy Society (ABS) recommendations for transperineal permanent brachytherapy of prostate cancer. Int J Radiat Oncol Biol Phys 1999; 44:789–99.

[10] American Joint Committee on Cancer. Prostate. AJCC cancer staging manual. 6th edition. New York: Springer; 2002. p. 309–16. Available at: www.cancer.gov/cancertopics/pdq/treatment/ prostate/HealthProfessional/page3#Reference3.15. Accessed August 23, 2006.

[11] Strang JG, Rubens DJ, Brasacchio RA, et al. Real-time US versus CT determination of pubic arch interference for brachytherapy. Radiology 2001; 219:387–93.

[12] Yu Y, Anderson LL, Li Z, et al. Permanent prostate seed implant brachytherapy: report of the American Association of Physicists in Medicine Task Group No. 64. Med Phys 1999;26:2054–76.

[13] Nag S, Ciezki JP, Cormack R, et al. Intraoperative planning and evaluation of permanent prostate brachytherapy: report of the American Brachytherapy Society. Int J Radiat Oncol Biol Phys 2001;51(5):1422–30.

[14] Yu Y, Zhang Y, Brasacchio RA, et al. Automated treatment planning engine for prostate seed

implant brachytherapy. Int J Radiat Oncol Biol Phys 1998;43:647–52.

[15] Nag S, Bice W, DeWyngaert K, et al. The American Brachytherapy Society recommendations for permanent prostate brachytherapy post-implant dosimetric analysis. Int J Radiat Oncol Biol Phys 2000;46:221–30.

[16] D'Amico AV, Cormack R, Tempany CM, et al. Real-time magnetic resonance image-guided interstitial brachytherapy in the treatment of select patients with clinically localized prostate cancer. Int J Radiat Oncol Biol Phys 1998;42: 507–15.

[17] D'Amico AV, Cormack RA, Tempany CM. MRI-guided diagnosis and treatment of prostate cancer. N Engl J Med 2001;344:776–7.

[18] Barnes AS, Tempany CM. Image-guided minimally invasive therapy. In: Richie JP, D'Amico A, editors. Urologic Oncology. Philadelphia: Elsevier; 2005. p. 113–31.

[19] Kurhanewicz J, Vigneron DB, Hricak H, et al. Three-dimensional H-1 MR spectroscopic imaging of the in situ human prostate with high

(0.24–0.7-cm3) spatial resolution. Radiology 1996;198:795–805.

[20] Bharatha A, Hirose M, Hata N, et al. Evaluation of three-dimensional finite element-based deformable registration of pre- and intraoperative prostate imaging. Med Phys 2001;28:2551–60.

[21] Barnes AS, Haker SJ, Mulkern RV, et al. Magnetic resonance spectroscopy-guided transperineal prostate biopsy and brachytherapy for recurrent prostate cancer. Urology 2005;66:1319.

[22] Kooy HM, Cormack RA, Mathiowitz G, et al. A software system for interventional magnetic resonance image-guided prostate brachytherapy. Comput Aided Surg 2000;5:401–13.

[23] Cormack RA, Kooy H, Tempany CM, et al. A clinical method for real-time dosimetric guidance of transperineal 125I prostate implants using interventional magnetic resonance imaging. Int J Radiat Oncol Biol Phys 2000;46:207–14.

[24] Cormack RA, Tempany CM, D'Amico AV. Optimizing target coverage by dosimetric feedback during prostate brachytherapy. Int J Radiat Oncol Biol Phys 2000;48:1245–9.

RADIOLOGIC
CLINICS
OF NORTH AMERICA

Radiol Clin N Am 44 (2006) 749–756

ELSEVIER
SAUNDERS

Imaging the Pediatric Prostate

Andrew Mong, MD*, Richard Bellah, MD

- Imaging techniques
- Embryology and development
- Congenital lesions
  Utricle and müllerian duct cysts
  Congenital polyps
- *Prune-belly syndrome*
- *Anorectal malformations*
- *Neoplasms*
- *Inflammatory diseases*
- Summary
- References

The prostate gland is not often the target of imaging in children but may be imaged during investigation of symptoms related to the lower genitourinary tract such as hematuria, urinary retention, dysuria, and incontinence or during an evaluation for suspected congenital anomalies. In this article, the authors outline the imaging techniques used to evaluate the pediatric prostate and discuss the congenital and neoplastic conditions that may be encountered.

Imaging techniques

Ultrasound is the initial diagnostic modality of choice to evaluate the pediatric lower urinary tract. A 5- to 7-MHz transducer is used transabdominally and, when high-resolution imaging is required for problem solving, a 7- to 12-MHz transducer may be used transperineally. The pediatric prostate is visualized through a full bladder as a hypoechoic, elliptically shaped, soft tissue structure at the bladder base (Fig. 1).

The prostatic urethra is not normally demonstrated by ultrasound, and is better evaluated by fluoroscopic voiding cystourethrography (VCUG), which is performed by inserting an 8F feeding tube through the urethra into the bladder with sterile technique, infusing radiographic contrast material into the urinary bladder, and imaging the urethra during voiding, preferably after the catheter has been removed. A retrograde urethrogram may also be performed if the bladder cannot be catheterized and may help to opacify a prostatic utricle or a fistula not visualized with VCUG due to the higher pressure generated during a retrograde injection.

MR imaging defines the cross-sectional anatomy of the prostate with greater tissue differentiation than CT. The prostate has homogeneous signal intensity on MR imaging that is isointense to muscle on T1-weighted images and iso- to hyperintense to muscle on T2-weighted images before puberty (Fig. 2). After puberty, the signal characteristics resemble those of the adult prostate.

Embryology and development

Development of the prostate begins at approximately 10 weeks of gestation. Vesicourethral components of the cloaca and a portion of the urogenital sinus contribute to the formation of the prostatic urethra. Under the influence of testosterone from adjacent mesenchyme, a cluster of prostatic evaginations from the prostatic urethra form at least five solid prostatic cords that develop lumina and acini. The surrounding mesenchyme

Department of Radiology, The Children's Hospital of Philadelphia, University of Pennsylvania School of Medicine, 34th and Civic Center Blvd, Philadelphia, PA 19104, USA
* Corresponding author.
E-mail address: mong@email.chop.edu (A. Mong).

doi:10.1016/j.rcl.2006.07.007

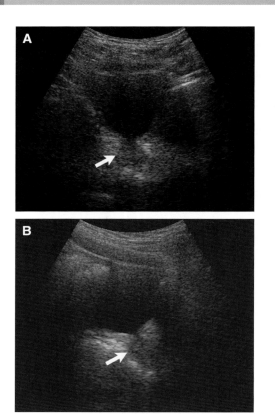

Fig. 1. (A) Transverse and (B) sagittal ultrasound images of a normal prostate (*arrows*) in a 4-year-old boy.

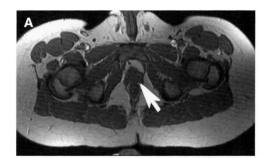

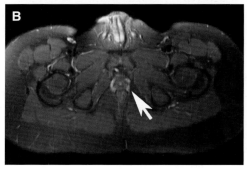

Fig. 2. (A) Axial T1-weighted and (B) fat-saturated axial T2-weighted MR images of normal prostate (*arrows*) in an 11-year-old prepubertal patient being evaluated for sacroiliitis.

contributes smooth muscle and connective tissue [1,2].

The verumontanum, a round protrusion on the posterior wall of the prostatic urethra, forms from components of the urogenital sinus and the caudally fused müllerian ducts. There is controversy concerning the origin of the prostatic utricle, a blind-ending sac that opens centrally into the prostatic urethra through the verumontanum. Originally described as a remnant of the fused müllerian ducts, histologic evidence suggests that it develops from the urogenital sinus as the müllerian ducts regress [3].

Between infancy and puberty, glandular tissues differentiate within the prostate, but lobar anatomy is not well defined, which may account for why it is not often easily seen with cross-sectional imaging. The prostate matures and grows in size during the 13th to 14th year, reaching adult size and development by 12 to 18 years [4]. Sonographic volume of the prostate ranges from 0.4 cm³ to 5.2 cm³ (mean, 1.2 cm³) in boys ranging in age from 7 months to 13.5 years [5]. This

measurement increases to 4.5 cm (transverse) × 3 cm (anterior posterior) × 4 cm (cephalocaudad), with a volume range from 12 to 20 cm³ in a young adult [6].

Congenital lesions

Utricle and müllerian duct cysts

The utricle is commonly seen on imaging studies and likely a normal finding when small. Enlarged utricles may be seen in conjunction with hypospadias, Down syndrome, imperforate anus, posterior urethral valves, prune-belly syndrome, and male pseudohermaphroditism [7,8]. An enlarged utricle (greater than 1 cm) or megautricle (much greater than 1 cm) may serve as a site of infection or stone formation secondary to urine stasis, may cause compression of the bladder neck and result in obstructive uropathy, or may be clinically silent. Müllerian duct cysts, in contradistinction, do not communicate with the urethra. They may occur anywhere along the path of müllerian duct regression and are not associated with other anomalies. The histologic origin of müllerian duct cysts is debated because a series of surgical specimens demonstrated epithelial lining identical to that of the prostatic utricle, with no epithelial evidence that they were a "remnant" of the regressed müllerian ducts [9].

Ultrasound of an enlarged prostatic utricle and a müllerian duct cyst reveals an anechoic cystic cavity behind the bladder. If the cyst is complicated or infected, there may hypoechoic debris. Echogenic shadowing stones may also be identified. Fluoroscopic evaluation with VCUG or retrograde urethrogram may be necessary to identify a connection with the posterior urethra to distinguish between a prostatic utricle and a müllerian duct cyst. On MR imaging, both anomalies are seen as T2 hyperintense cystic lesions posterior to the prostatic urethra (Fig. 3).

Congenital polyps

Congenital polyps of the prostatic urethra are hamartomatous lesions arising from the verumontanum, likely secondary to a developmental error of invagination rather than evagination of the primitive prostatic cords. They may present with dysuria, hematuria, enuresis, or urinary retention. The polyps may appear as small filling defects in the posterior urethra on VCUG and retrograde urethrogram or may be pedunculated, appearing in the bladder neck [10]. Ultrasound may reveal intraluminal spherical tissue at the bladder base if the polyp migrates into the bladder during the examination (Fig. 4). Smooth muscle hypertrophy of the bladder wall or dilation of the upper tracts may also be seen on the ultrasound examination, secondary to lower tract obstruction caused by the polyp.

Prune-belly syndrome

Prune-belly syndrome comprises the triad of cryptorchidism, abdominal wall muscle deficiency (giving the wrinkled "prune-belly" appearance), and urinary tract abnormalities. Prostatic hypoplasia is a central feature, with an increase in connective tissue and a decrease in smooth muscle within the prostate and throughout the urinary tract. The etiology of these findings is hypothesized to be secondary to (1) an arrest in primitive mesodermal development that fails to induce formation of the prostate or (2) an in utero urethral obstruction

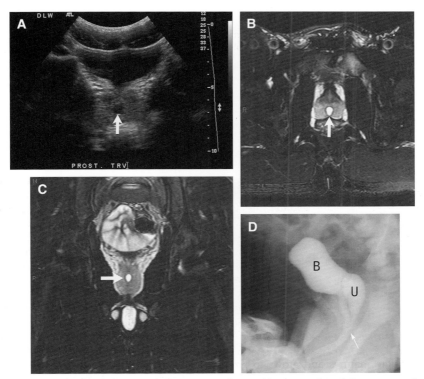

Fig. 3. Incidental prostatic utricle discovered during a work-up of hypertension. (*A*) Transverse image through the bladder base shows an anechoic structure (*arrow*) centered in the prostate. Axial T2-weighted MR image (*B*) and coronal T2-weighted image (*C*) show a well-defined hyperintense structure (*arrows*) corresponding to a prostatic utricle. (*D*) VCUG of a different patient who had hypospadias shows the connection of a utricle (*U*) to the prostatic urethra. B, urinary bladder.

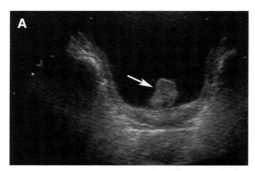

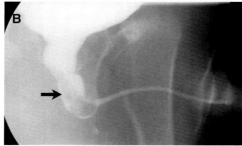

Fig. 4. (A) Transverse pelvic ultrasound image of a 3-year-old boy who had urinary retention shows a polyp (*arrow*) at the bladder base. (B) VCUG of the same patient shows the polyp located in the proximal urethra (*arrow*).

causing a distended bladder that secondarily induces pressure atrophy of the prostate [11,12]. Ectasia of the urinary tract from the renal pelves to the prostatic urethra is a hallmark of prune-belly syndrome. VCUG may reveal a funnel-shaped bladder neck and dilation of the posterior urethra,

thought to be secondary to the prostatic hypoplasia (Fig. 5).

Anorectal malformations

Anorectal malformations represent a spectrum of complex anomalies that often include fistula formation and atretic distal bowel with rectal pouch. They are classified as high, intermediate, or low, depending on the relationship of the rectal pouch to the puborectal sling. Fistula formation from bowel above the atretic segment in boys may be to the bladder, urethra, perineum, or cloaca.

Rectal agenesis may be associated with a rectourinary fistula, which may be high (at the level of the bladder, internal sphincter, or prostatic urethra) or intermediate (at the level of the bulbar urethra). Low anorectal malformations are typically anocutaneous and do not involve the urethra, although an anourethral-cutaneous fistula has been reported [13].

The prostate may be maldeveloped in association with a rectourinary fistula. Commonly, a rectourinary fistula occurs at the prostatic urethra at the level of the verumontanum, with the prostate gland developing above and lateral to the fistula but not caudal to it. When the fistula arises from the bladder, the prostate is rudimentary and forms around the fistula's orifice. When the fistula connects to the bulbar urethra, the prostate gland develops normally [14].

Clinical inspection of the perineum combined with urinalysis may provide surgeons with accurate classification of the anorectal malformations in 80% to 90% of cases, allowing treatment decisions to be made such as primary anastamosis for low

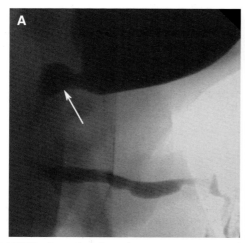

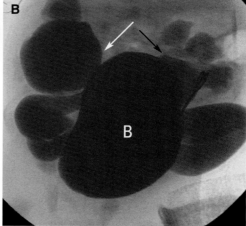

Fig. 5. VCUG of a male infant demonstrates ectasia of the prostatic urethra (A) and reflux into markedly ectatic ureters and collecting systems (*arrows*) bilaterally (B). B, bladder.

anorectal malformations versus initial diverting colostomy for high or intermediate lesions [15]. Prone cross-table radiographs, traditionally used to infer the level of the levator sling in relation to an air-distended rectal pouch, are inaccurate because the puborectalis muscle may ascend 2 to 3 cm during crying [16].

When there is clinical doubt as to the level of the malformation, MR imaging has been advocated as a means of defining the rectal pouch in relation to the external anal sphincter. Two axial planes may be defined with MR imaging: one that includes the symphysis pubis and the coccyx ("PC" plain) and one defined by the ischial rami ("I" plain). The PC plain normally includes the prostate and the puborectalis muscle, and the I plain normally includes the external anal sphincter. The rectal pouch may be distended with meconium and demonstrate bright T1 signal; it is considered high if it is above the PC plane, intermediate if it is included in the PC plane but not the I plane, and low if it is included in the I plane [17,18]. The presence of a fistula, however, may be better demonstrated with VCUG than with MR imaging (Fig. 6) [18].

Neoplasms

Rhabdomyosarcoma

Rhabdomyosarcoma is a tumor of skeletal muscle differentiation. Genitourinary sites are second in frequency (25%) after head and neck (35%), with the prostate and bladder representing 5% of all cases [19]. Other genitourinary sites of tumor origin in the male patient include the testicles, paratesticular tissues, penis, and perineum [20]. Rhabdomyosarcoma is the most common

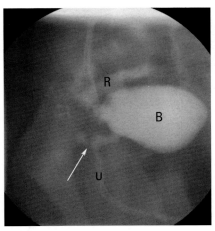

Fig. 6. VCUG of a 1-month-old infant who had imperforate anus demonstrates a fistula (*arrow*) from the prostatic urethra (U) to the rectum (R). B, bladder.

pediatric malignancy of the prostate, and patients may present with gross hematuria and symptoms of urinary tract/bladder outlet obstruction. Primary chemotherapy followed by radical surgery of the prostate or bladder may allow total tumor resection and yield high cure rates of approximately 80% [21]. Bladder salvage is only possible in the absence of residual disease.

The features of rhabdomyosarcoma on ultrasound are varied, with the mass presenting as heterogeneous or homogeneously hypoechoic. Blood flow within the mass may help distinguish it from other entities such as cyst, blood clot, or abscess. The site of origin of the tumor may be difficult to determine with ultrasound and may be better distinguished with CT or MR imaging, which may also identify enlarged regional lymph nodes (greater than 1 cm). MR imaging may be able to detect bladder wall invasion, with T2-weighted images demonstrating the higher–signal intensity tumor extending into the lower–signal intensity wall. T1-weighted images may demonstrate invasion into perivesical and perirectal fat (Fig. 7).

Miscellaneous tumors

Patients who have neurofibromatosis type I are at elevated risk for developing rhabdomyosarcoma of the prostate but may also develop prostatic masses secondary to neurofibromas or malignant schwannomas [22,23]. Pelvic plexiform neurofibromas display intermediate signal intensity on T1-weighted imaging (slightly higher than skeletal muscle) and high signal intensity on T2-weighted imaging (Fig. 8).

Other pediatric prostatic tumors are extremely rare. Leukemic infiltration demonstrates similar MR imaging features to lymphoma, with hypovascularity and only mild contrast enhancement.

Prostate carcinoma has been reported in 15 children younger than 17 years [24]. Imaging findings of prostate carcinoma in the pediatric population have not been described.

Primary carcinoid involving the prostate in a patient who had multiple endocrine neoplasia IIb has been reported [25].

Inflammatory diseases

Inflammation of the pediatric prostate is rare. Chronic prostatitis may be secondary to abnormal voiding conditions, with resultant high voiding pressures. Chronic reflux of urine into the prostate may cause large calcifications (Fig. 9) and be associated with chronic prostatitis or chronic pelvic pain syndrome in young men [26].

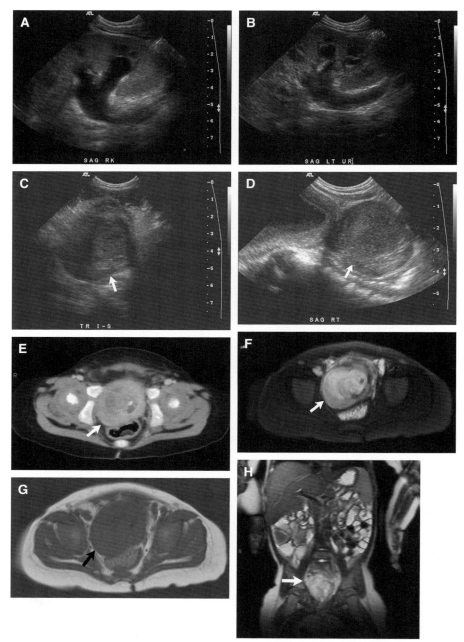

Fig. 7. Eight-month-old infant presenting with urinary retention. (A, B) Ultrasound demonstrates bilateral hy-dronephosis. Sagittal (C) and axial (D) images through the bladder neck demonstrate a mass (arrows) replac-ing the prostate with dilation of a debris-filled bladder. Postcontrast axial CT (E), axial T2-weighted (F), axial T1-weighted (G), and coronal T2-weighted (H) images demonstrate the extent of the rhabdomyosarcoma (arrows).

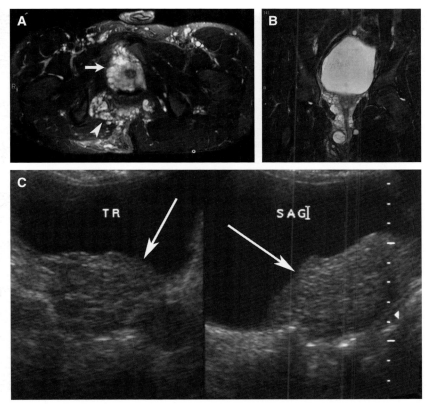

Fig. 8. Axial (*A*) and coronal (*B*) short tau inversion recovery images demonstrate multiple small neurofibromas within the prostate (*arrow*) and surrounding the prostate and in the subcutaneous tissues (*arrowhead*). (*C*) The prostate of a different patient who had neurofibromatosis demonstrates contour abnormality from small neurofibromas (*arrows*).

Summary

Pathology of the pediatric prostate is rare. Ultrasound and VCUG are useful for initial evaluation of congenital and neoplastic disorders of the prostate. MR imaging and CT are useful in delineating more detailed anatomy before surgical planning and in determining the organ of origin in a patient who has a large pelvic mass.

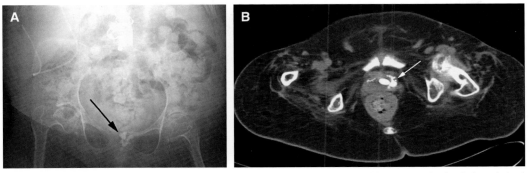

Fig. 9. Plain radiograph (*A*) and axial CT image (*B*) of the pelvis in a 17-year-old patient who had chronic hydrocephalus. Large dystrophic calcifications are noted in the midline of the pelvis (*arrows*), which also demonstrates a dysplastic osteopenic gracile pelvis and coxa vara of the right hip. The calcifications are confirmed to be in the prostate with CT.

References

[1] Cunha GR, Ricke W, Thomson A, et al. Hormonal, cellular, and molecular regulation of normal and neoplastic prostatic development. J Steroid Biochem Mol Biol 2004;92:221–36.

[2] Larsen WJ. Human embryology. New York: Churchill Livingstone; 1993.

[3] Shapiro E, Huang H, McFadden DE, et al. The prostatic utricle is not a Mullerian duct remnant: immunohistochemical evidence for a distinct urogenital sinus origin. J Urol 2004;172: 1753–64.

[4] Zondek T, Zondek LH. The fetal and neonatal prostate. In: Goland M, editor. Normal and abnormal growth of the prostate. Springfield (IL): Thomas; 1975. p. 5–28.

[5] Ingram S, Hollman AS, Azmy AFA. Ultrasound evaluation of the paediatric prostate. Br J Urol 1994;74:601–3.

[6] Shapiro E, Hartanto V, Perlman EJ, et al. Morphometric analysis of pediatric and nonhyperplastic prostate glands. Evidence that BPH isnot a unique stromal process. Prostate 1997;33:177–82.

[7] Currarino G. Urethro-ejaculatory reflux during cystourethrography in 25 children. J Urol 1993; 150:446–51.

[8] Currarino G. Large prostatic utricles and related structures, urogenital sinus and other forms of urethrovaginal confluence. J Urol 1986;136: 1270–9.

[9] Kato H, Hayama M, Furuya S, et al. Anatomical and histological studies of so-called Mullerian duct cyst. Int J Urol 2005;12:465–8.

[10] Aragona F, Di Tonno F, Tuccitto G, et al. Congenital polyp of the prostatic urethra: report on 2 cases. Urol Int 1988;43:113–7.

[11] Volmar KE, Fritsch MK, Perlman EJ, et al. Patterns of congenital lower urinary tract obstructive uropathy: relation to abnormal prostate and bladder development and the prune belly syndrome. Pediatr Dev Pathol 2001;4:467–72.

[12] Popek EJ, Tyson RW, Miller GJ, et al. Prostate development in prune belly syndrome (PBS) and posterior urethral valves (PUV): etiology of PBS—lower urinary tract obstruction or primary mesenchymal defect? Pediatr Pathol 1991;11: 1–29.

[13] Kumar V, Rao PL, Vepakomma D. Low anorectal malformation associated with 'ano-urethrocutaneous' fistula. Pediatr Surg Int 2005;21: 829–30.

[14] Stephens FD, Smith ED, Hutson JM. Congenital anomalies of the urinary and genital tracts. Oxford: Oxford, UK: Isis Medical Media Ltd.; 1996.

[15] Pena A. Management of anorectal malformations in the newborn period. World J Surg 1993;17: 385–92.

[16] Berdon WE, Baker TV, Santulli TV, et al. The radiologic evaluation of imperforate anus. Radiology 1968;90:466–71.

[17] Sato Y, Pringle KC, Bergman RA, et al. Congenital anorectal anomalies: MR imaging. Radiology 1988;168:157–62.

[18] McHugh K. The role of radiology in children with anorectal anomalies; with particular emphasis on MRI. Eur J Radiol 1998;26:194–9.

[19] Nigro KG, MacLennan GT. Rhabdomyosarcoma of the bladder and prostate. J Urol 2005;173: 1365.

[20] Geoffrey A, Agrons GA, Wagner BJ. From the archives of the AFIP: genitourinary rhabdomyosarcoma in children. Radiographics 1997;17: 919–37.

[21] Filipas D, Fisch M, Stein R, et al. Rhabdomyosarcoma of the bladder, prostate or vagina: the role of surgery. BJU Int 2004;93:125–9.

[22] Rames RA, Smith MT. Malignant peripheral nerve sheath tumor of the prostate: a rare manifestation of neurofibromatosis type 1. J Urol 1999;162:165–6.

[23] Chung AK, Michels V, Poland GA, et al. Neurofibromatosis with involvement of the prostate gland. Urology 1996;47:448–51.

[24] Shimada H, Misugi K, Sasaki Y, et al. Carcinoma of the prostate in childhood and adolescence: report of a case and review of the literature. Cancer 1980;46:2534–42.

[25] Whelan T, Gatfield CT, Robertson S, et al. Primary carcinoid of the prostate in conjunction with multiple endocrine neoplasia IIb in a child. J Urol 1995;153:1080–2.

[26] Geramoutos I, Gyftopoulos K, Perimenis P, et al. Clinical correlation of prostatic lithiasis with chronic pelvic pain syndromes in young adults. Eur Urol 2004;45:333–8.

RADIOLOGIC CLINICS OF NORTH AMERICA

Radiol Clin N Am 44 (2006) 757–761

ELSEVIER SAUNDERS

Index

Note: Page numbers of article titles are in **boldface** type.

doi:10.1016/S0033-8389(06)00087-X

Moving?

Make sure your subscription moves with you!

To notify us of your new address, find your **Clinics Account Number** (located on your mailing label above your name), and contact customer service at:

E-mail: elspcs@elsevier.com

800-654-2452 (subscribers in the U.S. & Canada)
407-345-4000 (subscribers outside of the U.S. & Canada)

Fax number: 407-363-9661

Elsevier Periodicals Customer Service
6277 Sea Harbor Drive
Orlando, FL 32887-4800

*To ensure uninterrupted delivery of your subscription, please notify us at least 4 weeks in advance of move.